D0268256

List of tables and figures

Tables

Figures

Contents

Acknowledgements

We would like to thank a number of people who helped with the research that underpins this book:

- Stuart Anderson and Stephen Peckham of the National Institute for Health Research (NIHR) Service Delivery and Organisation (SDO) Programme that funded the research.
- Jane Martin contributed to the literature review and undertook early drafts of two chapters.
- Erin Withers, Layla Branicki and Kwaku Dako provided library and bibliographic help.
- Yvonne Field provided secretarial help with the manuscript.

The SDO Project Advisory Group and others gave initial and continuing advice throughout the project and a number of them read through an earlier draft:

- Cynthia Bower, Chief Executive, Quality Care Commission.
- Elisabeth Buggins, Chair, West Midlands Strategic Health Authority.
- Sophia Christie, Chief Executive, NHS Birmingham East and North PCT (Primary Care Trust).
- David Cox, Chair, NHS South Birmingham (Primary Care Trust).
- Bernard Crump, Chief Executive, NHS Institute for Innovation and Improvement.
- Keith Grint, Institute of Governance and Public Management, Warwick Business School.
- Emma Hawkridge, Press Office, SDO.
- Liam Hughes, National Advisor for Healthy Communities, Improvement and Development Agency for Local Government.
- Sue James, Chief Executive, Walsall Hospital Trust.
- Jake Lyne, Consultant Clinical Psychologist.
- Gerry McSorley, Head of Board Development, NHS Institute for Innovation and Improvement.
- Peter Spurgeon, Warwick Medical School.
- Tamar Thompson, Director of Nursing and Workforce, West Midlands Strategic Health Authority.
- Heinrich Volmink, Health Improvement Practitioner, West Glasgow Community Health & Care Partnership.

CHAPTER 1

Introducing leadership

Writing, advice and training on leadership are growing at such a rate that the 'field' of leadership is better described as a tropical jungle. The plants (ideas, books, practices) are growing very vigorously, with more information being produced than could be read by a single person in a lifetime. Theories, concepts and ideas about leadership create such a thick undergrowth that it can be hard to hack your way through. It is not that any particular theory is difficult; it is just that there are so many of them, competing for the sunlight. A troupe of guru monkeys is chattering and screaming in the high canopy of the forest. You crane your neck up to catch sight of them, but they have just leapt on to the next tree. Exotic theory birds swoop past, with dazzling plumage, but they don't stay put long enough to enable you to examine them closely. Down at your feet on the jungle floor, there are snakes that may appear innocuous but can be deadly. There is a lot of vegetation but it is hard to work out which is nutritious and which is poisonous.

Grint (2005a) notes that while we have a surfeit of information about leadership, there is much less in the way of understanding. Burns (1978) wrote that "leadership is one of the most observed and least understood phenomena on earth" (p 2). So, how does one survive and thrive in this jungle? This book aims to provide a compass, a map and a naturalist's guide to help find a path through the undergrowth, and to enjoy the journey.

The compass is our attempt to provide strategic direction and clarity of purpose by offering concepts and theories that may help to make sense of the complexities of leadership talk and action. The map is the analytical framework, developed by the authors on the basis of the general leadership literature, and here applied to healthcare, to provide an orientation to the landscape, and to help to hack out a clear path through the jungle. The map is an analytical framework not a single theory, because the book covers a wide range of leadership phenomena (leaders, leadership, contexts, outcomes and so on) and in each of these areas particular theories may be relevant and useful. But the map provides an overview and a structure by which to analyse theory and practice. When you are feeling stuck – as a researcher in the literature or as a healthcare practitioner subjected to different exhortations or pressures about how to behave as a leader – then we hope that this map will help you, by being able to place theories in a framework, or conceptual structure.

This book will be of interest to all who exercise leadership in relation to healthcare. This includes those who have a formal leadership position in a healthcare organisation (for example, chief executive, clinical director, doctor, nurse manager) or those whose leadership is through influencing thinking and actions relevant to healthcare (for example, local government elected members and officers, patient groups).

At the strategic level this book will be of interest to board members, clinical directors, finance directors, senior managers and human resource (HR) professionals – and also health scrutiny members and officers in local government.

At the operational level, the book will be of interest to health professionals, such as doctors, nurses, pharmacists and other professions, in leading and influencing healthcare and improvements in healthcare.

The framework and the research evidence will also be of interest to policy-makers and policy advisors, and to health researchers, particularly those concerned with service delivery and organisation, with leadership and the evaluation of leadership development.

Finally, the map will be of generic interest to leadership researchers, whatever their field (jungle?) of study or the sector they are focused on. While the focus here is on healthcare, the book draws on insights, theories and evidence from the leadership field in general. The analytical framework is generic while the application (to healthcare) is specific.

We examine those aspects of the literature where there is an evidence base for ideas and practices about leadership and we aim to apply rigorous thinking to how such theories and ideas can be applied. 'Evidence-based' medicine has gained considerable ground over recent years, and there is a growing interest in evidence-based management as well (Walshe and Rundall, 2001; Tranfield et al, 2003; Rousseau, 2006). The fact that leadership studies are multidisciplinary and located in the social sciences and humanities rather than medical science means that the evidence base for leadership will always be different from, and more open to, value-laden debate than would occur in subjects covered in medical science. Evidence in this field is sometimes more like evidence in a court of law than in a laboratory – subject to dialogue, challenge and refutation. This discursive debate is part of the process of evaluation of the evidence (Morgan, 1997; Flyberg, 2001; Marsh and Stoker, 2002; Moses and Knutsen, 2007). Having a clear sense of which leadership ideas and practices are rooted in theory and evidence, and which are more speculative or normative, can be very helpful for leaders surrounded by conflicting advice, or being urged to behave in particular ways because it is fashionable. Having a clear compass and map of the terrain of leadership will help to avoid at least some of the pitfalls, fallacies and fantasies about leadership.

The literature used for this enquiry into the evidence base for public leadership, and specifically leadership in healthcare, came from several sources. First, we carried out an examination of the recent academic literature on leadership in healthcare organisations and networks. Second, we asked for key recommendations for articles, books and reports from 43 academic experts in the field of leadership and/or healthcare. Third, the authors drew on their wider knowledge of the leadership literature to introduce theories and ideas that are currently absent from the healthcare field but which have been established in other areas of leadership enquiry, and which have potential for the healthcare field. Fourth, we regularly tested and checked both our ideas and our writing with a range of healthcare practitioners, from a range of roles and disciplines, so that we could ensure that the ideas and the writing are accessible, practical and useful.

New look leadership – the height of fashion?

Leadership is currently a trendy topic (Storey, 2004; Grint, 2005a; Burke and Cooper, 2006; Jackson and Parry, 2008), with literally hundreds of new books and articles being published by the day. Google records 122 million references to leadership and 35.6 million to public leadership. 'Leadership' has replaced 'management' in some quarters as the fashionable language of business. The interest in leadership is particularly evident in the public sector (Hartley, 2010a). There has been a series of government policy papers asserting the importance of leadership in public service improvement, stemming from the influential Performance and Innovation Unit report of 2001 (Cabinet Office, 2001) and reflected in the titles of a number of White Papers. Dedicated leadership centres and programmes have been set up for particular public service sectors including central government, local government, schools, health, fire service, further education, higher education, police and the voluntary sector among others – and a Public Service Leadership Alliance (PSLA) set up to coordinate their efforts (Benington and Hartley, 2009).

Health is no exception to this trend, and 'better leadership' is seen as central to improving the quality of healthcare and the improvement of organisational processes. *The NHS plan* (DH, 2000) argued for more attention to be paid to leadership and the development of leaders and led to the establishment of the NHS Institute for Innovation and Improvement, which has a key stream of work on leadership development as well as improvement and innovation. More recently and very prominently, the Darzi report *Next stage review* (DH, 2008) places considerable emphasis on healthcare leadership, especially but not exclusively by clinicians, as the NHS tackles new challenges to improve health quality and care. From the opposite end of the argument, some of the high-profile media cases of lapses in professional care in the UK have, in part, been attributed to problems of leadership, as in the Bristol Royal Infirmary case, and in the Victoria Climbié case (although weakness in leadership is clearly not the whole story).

Although leadership is currently highlighted as one of the fashionable solutions to the complex challenges in healthcare (including the current financial crisis and threat of severe cutbacks in public expenditure), we think there are several reasons why leadership needs to be taken seriously as part of longer-term strategies for public service improvement and innovation. The profound restructuring of the ecological, political, economic, social and technological context is posing major new systemic challenges for governments and communities, and requires a Copernican revolution in mindsets as well as new patterns of action. Many of these issues (for example, climate change; care for an ageing population; crime and the fear of crime) are both complex and contested – there is no clear agreement about either the causes or the solutions to the problems. There are no ready-made technical solutions to these 'wicked' or 'adaptive' problems, and they often cannot be solved by a single profession or a single public service alone but require exploratory effort from a range of people, organisations and sectors.

There are therefore several reasons why leadership – both within the organisation and between organisations and across networks – needs to be taken seriously:

- There are many new challenges in healthcare, including changes in the kinds of illnesses to be confronted. For example, the major post-war curable diseases, such as measles and diphtheria, are largely conquered but instead chronic and multiple diseases associated with a larger elderly population, and chronic diseases due to lifestyle choices (such as obesity and smoking), are becoming more important. How can leadership be used to anticipate rather than just react to changes in demographic and disease profiles?
- There are new health goals. Partly because of the changing pattern of illness and also because of the longer-term pressures on budgets, 'predict and prevent' have become more important goals alongside 'treatment'. Health promotion not just sickness alleviation is now of

more concern. Healthcare in the community, not just in hospitals and clinics, is increasingly important. Public health may be moving back to the centre of health policy. Working with partner organisations becomes increasingly important. How can leadership be deployed to help shape these new goals, and to ensure that ideas are translated into more effective practices at the front-line of the NHS organisation, and between different partners?

- The expectations of patients, carers and communities are increasing with more widespread knowledge about health available via the internet, less deference towards professional and medical authority, and higher expectations of personalised and flexible care. What are the implications for healthcare organisations and their staff and how can leadership be used to ensure that these changes are seized as opportunities to innovate and improve the quality of healthcare?
- The new techniques and technologies emerging in healthcare require new ways of working both within and across teams, and with patients. Who can lead such changes and how might they be carried out?
- New approaches to self-sustaining continuous improvement, which rely as much on mobilising and motivating staff as on the techniques themselves, are being introduced. How can leaders support staff to make and sustain local problem-solving efforts in order to improve the service to the patient?
- The increasing emphasis on step-change innovation, and not just on continuous improvement, aims to improve safety, quality and efficiency in healthcare. How can leaders create the conditions for creative problem-solving and the taking of reasonable risks through innovation?
- The organisations of healthcare are changing – with not only new structures, such as Foundation Trusts, but also new cultures and ways of working. How might such changes be led?

These are just some of the reasons why leadership is important in healthcare. New paradigm thinking is helping to shift the emphasis away from a 'one best way' model of leadership towards thinking about a repertoire of different approaches and methods to be deployed according to the flow of change and the movement of the action. The arts of public leadership now have to include skills, for example, in deciding when to use hierarchies, markets or networks, and when to use exit, voice or loyalty, as part of the leadership repertoire (Benington, 2006).

The Warwick 6 C framework for thinking about leadership

> Leadership research has a narrow focus, and there has been little integration of findings from different approaches. (Yukl, 2006, p 445)

Much writing on leadership is very descriptive and anecdotal. For example, leadership manuals and books often begin with a set of prescriptive behaviours, competencies or qualities required of individual leaders, and some assertions about the impact that leadership can have on team or organisational performance. A lot of books and articles on leadership consist of lists of ideal traits or inspirational behaviours, divorced from both theory and context. Some may provide guidance principles of the 'do this, don't do that' kind. These tend, therefore, to be aspirational and prescriptive about the good qualities of leadership or the skills and behaviours that are shown by effective leaders. This has been described as the 'heroic' approach to leadership. Indeed, the illustrations of leadership qualities and behaviours are often derived from heroic personalities and heroic situations – arctic explorers, political leaders in war or crises, business leaders turning around major companies on the brink of bankruptcy. Such approaches may be particularly appealing in the health service, where the heroic consultant or doctor (and their sibling the heroic manager) have been applauded for their successes. In such narratives the focus is generally on the leader's characteristics as an individual, rather than on the context or the other actors and partners in the process.

This simplistic individualistic perspective in much leadership writing means that there are relatively few conceptual frameworks to help analyse leadership as a dynamic and contested process within a complex adaptive 'whole system'. Such frameworks are few and far between, but they are very important if leaders and potential leaders are to take an overview of the field and to have a compass and map for their own practices and reflections.

Storey (2004, p 341), to take one helpful example, presents a leadership framework based on an interlocking set of factors – the impact of both the industry or organisational context, and the ideological context, on leadership, the perceived need for leadership, the behavioural requirements of the leader and leadership development methods. His framework also includes a consideration of outcomes in terms of unit performance, and evaluations by a range of stakeholders.

Yukl (2006) is another writer who proposes an 'integrating conceptual framework', but one based on predicting the behaviour of the individual leader from their traits, behaviours and power resources, and from those of 'followers'. This is a view of leadership based in individual and small group influence processes and is valuable as far as it goes but it provides little sense of an organisational or institutional context to understanding leadership or of how leadership frames meanings and purposes. Heifetz's (1994) theory of leadership includes a number of features that constitute an integrative framework, although he does not himself make this claim. We return to the work of Heifetz at several points in this book.

The lack of satisfactory integrating theories of leadership has led the authors to develop the Warwick Six C Leadership Framework, which provides a lens through which to scrutinise the leadership literature and to provide an overview that takes into account key elements affecting leadership processes and outcomes. This is shown in Figure 1.1 below. The framework is also the basis on which the book is structured. This framework is relevant to leadership in general, although in this book we are using it to examine specifically leadership in healthcare.

Figure 1.1: The Warwick Six C Leadership Framework

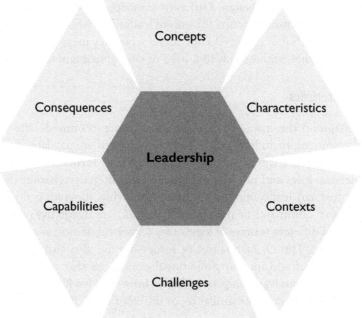

Copyright: John Benington and Jean Hartley

An analytical framework, as noted earlier, is not a theory. It does not seek to explain phenomena (as theory aims to) but rather offers a structure for categorising and interpreting aspects of leadership. In this way, the framework is able to group particular aspects of leadership studies together in order to illuminate knowledge and findings in ways that are conceptually appealing and practically useful. The grouping of ideas under different aspects of leadership reduces the confusion caused by the plethora of perspectives and ideas, and also helps to indicate where research, knowledge or practice is lacking. It can also clarify relationships between different elements of leadership.

The Warwick Six C Leadership Framework is used, first, to examine different dimensions of leadership and, second, in the last chapter, to consider the implications for leadership development. It has six elements in its structure, and each element is covered in a single chapter.

Concepts

In Chapter 2, this book examines the different concepts that are used to define and explain leadership, noting that the definition of leadership influences the ways in which leadership behaviours, processes and outcomes are viewed. The different approaches to leadership taken by different authors have an impact on the questions and the use of evidence about leadership. Different concepts mean that different authors emphasise particular features of leadership while downplaying other aspects. Some authors do not define what they mean by leadership in their studies, which leads to a haze of conceptual ambiguity.

Characteristics

In Chapter 3, the characteristics of leadership are examined – the roles and resources, including power resources, which are available to the leadership. The chapter explores how far and why formal and informal leadership roles and processes are similar or different; whether direct (face-to-face) leadership and indirect leadership (operating through a chain of command or distributed network) are distinctive; and the impact of different sources of legitimacy (expertise, democratic election and so on). The characteristics of leadership are also shaped by the organisational and inter-organisational conditions that may support, enhance or limit leadership. In addition, how far is leadership of inter-organisational networks similar to, or different from, the leadership of discrete organisations?

Contexts

In Chapter 4, themes and questions about context are identified, because the context (for example, political and economic context, policy context, organisational context) both creates opportunities for and places constraints on action and is also a source of potential leverage for leaders. In particular, healthcare raises critical questions about the importance of the political, economic, social and institutional context, which has perhaps been underplayed in many analyses of healthcare leadership. This also raises questions as to how far the sector/industry, institutional or organisational context has been sufficiently examined in accounts of leadership more generally. In addition, there is more work to be done to understand how leaders 'read' the changing context and scan, interpret and articulate the nature of the wider environment for the group, organisation or network. Context is critical to understanding the processes and consequences of leadership.

Challenges

In Chapter 5, the challenges of leadership – which concern the principal purposes, goals or aims that leaders and leadership attempt to address – are explored. These challenges are crucial to leadership and it can be argued that 'the primary task' or public value goals of leadership are central to understanding leadership effectiveness, although not all leadership studies address this question of purpose. The interest in 'new leadership' (for example, charismatic leadership, transformational leadership) brought the value of 'vision' back into leadership studies. In fact, the purposes of leadership often go beyond vision into the goals, values and aims of leadership. How are purposes formulated, articulated and debated? The complex context of healthcare makes this a particularly fertile site for the exploration and contestation of purposes by different stakeholders. In particular, for public services such as healthcare, there is also the question of assessing whether or not the leadership purposes contribute to, or detract from, the creation of the wider public good or public value, or whether they overly focus on organisational outputs (Benington and Moore, 2010).

Capabilities

Chapter 6 examines capabilities. These are the qualities (for example, traits, skills, abilities, mindsets, behaviours) that are thought to distinguish 'leaders' from 'followers' and/or to contribute to successful or effective leadership. The chapter explores a variety of frameworks, from trait and style theory to behaviour theory and competency frameworks, and looks at this not only in terms of individuals but also of groups such as teams, boards and partnerships. The chapter explores in more depth recent interest in emotional intelligence and leadership with political awareness, before looking at the evidence about the popular transformational and transactional leadership theory, and then post-transformational theory.

Consequences

In Chapter 7, the review examines the consequences of leadership, rigorously questioning the extent to which the claims of a link between leadership and performance are justified, both in terms of evidence of causation and also because of attributional processes. Evidence of impact is then explored, by using the public value chain (covering inputs, activities, partnerships, outputs, user satisfaction and outcomes) and emphasising the need to consider the contribution to the common good not just contribution to organisational or network effectiveness.

Leadership development

Finally, in Chapter 8, the book reuses the analytical framework but this time placing 'leadership development' not 'leadership' in the centre of the diagram. This chapter is about the ideas and the evidence for types of leadership development and how effective they are found to be. The analytical framework is re-employed because the same issues of analytical clarity dog the leadership development literature. How leadership is conceptualised will influence the kinds of leadership development that are promoted. The analysis of the characteristics of leadership will shape leadership development programmes – leadership development for chief executives or clinicians may need different emphases than leadership development for nurses or board members, for example. Leadership development cannot be based on 'one size fits all'. Leadership development requires analysis of the contexts of leadership otherwise the design of opportunities and programmes will lack realistic preparation for participants. Learning to read context is a key leadership skill, so how do leadership development programmes prepare for this? Similarly, without an analysis of the challenges of leadership, now and in the future, there could be inadequate or inappropriate development opportunities for healthcare leaders. Capability models often lie at the heart of leadership development programmes but there can be dangers if capabilities are not seen as interacting with context and challenges. The question in relation to the consequences element of the model is how can one tell whether leadership development programmes make a difference? Is the expenditure on leadership development justified not only in terms of individual learning but also organisational improvement? This requires understanding of the varied consequences of leadership and of different evaluation frameworks. Each of these issues will be explored further in the following chapters.

Policy and practice implications:

- Understanding leadership is an increasingly important task for healthcare policy-makers and managers as the goals and context of healthcare in the UK become more complex.
- Leadership is a very fashionable topic in the public sector, so there are grounds for some scepticism. But leadership is not just a passing fad, and it is worth considering whether and how it can contribute to healthcare improvement.
- Much leadership literature focuses on heroic individuals but there is a need to go beyond that to consider a wider range of influences on leadership as part of a complex dynamic system, including concepts, characteristics, contexts, challenges, capabilities and consequences.
- Using the Warwick Six C Leadership Framework (Figure 1.1) will help to analyse leadership in a more rounded way, increasing the opportunity to be effective in healthcare settings.

CHAPTER 2

Leadership concepts

In this chapter:

We note that there are many and varied definitions and ideas about what leadership is and we explore the different interpretations. The chapter examines three main approaches to conceptualising leadership, in terms of a focus on the person, the position or the processes. It is valuable to be aware of these different concepts of leadership in thinking about leadership otherwise talk and action may be at cross-purposes. Each emphasises different facets of leadership and may be incomplete on its own.

Figure 2.1: The concepts of leadership

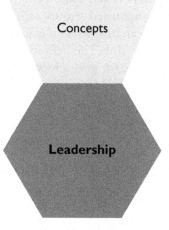

This chapter examines the first segment of the Warwick Six C Leadership Framework set out in the previous chapter. So, here we examine leadership concepts. Why use the plural (that is, concepts) rather than the singular (that is, concept) when discussing leadership? There are very many definitions of leadership provided by academics and the term is used in myriad ways in everyday speech. Furthermore, the term has changed in emphasis or approach over time, as overviews of the history of leadership research show (for example, Storey, 2004; Parry and Bryman, 2006).

These different emphases could be the basis for considerable confusion unless we unpack and examine the various ways in which the term leadership is defined and used. Grint (2000) argues that the term is 'multifaceted'. Many writers avoid the complexity entirely and fail to indicate what they mean by leadership!

What is meant by the term leadership?

An early definition of leadership from the 1950s is still helpful:

> Leadership may be considered as the process (act) of influencing the activities of an organized group in its efforts towards goal setting and goal achievement. (Stogdill, 1950, p 3)

This has a number of elements – it views leadership as a social and relational process of influence occurring within a group. So, leadership is seen here not just in terms of individual characteristics but about what happens between leaders and those being influenced. Stogdill's definition is about an organised group, although there may be arguments that leadership can have wider impacts, for example, outside as well as inside the organisation. The definition also links leadership to purposes – goal setting and/or goal achievement. This suggests that the work that the group aims to do together is central to the definition. This definition is focused not on a person but on a process (influence).

Other definitions emphasise these features, to a greater or lesser degree. For example:

- "leadership over human beings is exercised when persons with certain motives and purposes mobilize, in competition or conflict with others, institutional, political, psychological, and other resources so as to arouse, engage and satisfy the motives of followers" (Burns, 1978, p 18);
- "leadership is realized in the process whereby one or more individuals succeed in attempting to frame and define the reality of others" (Smircich and Morgan, 1982, p 258);
- "the process of inducing others to take action towards a common goal" (Locke, 1991, p 2);
- "mobilising people to tackle tough problems" (Heifetz, 1994, p 15).

These definitions are drawn from a range of fields where leadership has been observed (managerial, organisational, political) and are seen as generically relevant.

In the health field, Goodwin argues for a definition of leadership based on a systems–wide view:

> Leadership is a dynamic process of pursuing a vision for change in which the leader is supported by two main groups: followers within the leader's own organization, and influential players and other organizations in the leader's wider, external environment. (Goodwin, 2006, p 22)

These definitions vary substantially – whether the definition focuses on the purposes or goals, or whether it focuses on the social dynamics; whether the focus is the group, the organisation or the social system; whether the intention is to satisfy followers or to engage them in difficult problem-solving (tough problems). They do have in common the idea of influence between human beings, with particular purposes to be achieved.

Perspectives on leadership

In this chapter we use a threefold typology of leadership concepts to reflect the relative emphases placed on:

- the personal qualities of the leader;
- the leadership positions in the organisation;
- the social processes and interactions of leadership.

Hartley and Allison (2000) have conceptualised leadership from the three perspectives of 'person, position and process'. These three approaches are shown in Table 2.1.

Personal qualities of the leader

Research on the personal characteristics of leaders abounds and Yukl (2006) provides a good overview. Early work tried to find the personality types or innate personal characteristics (traits) that were associated with leadership, but this work largely foundered both because the list of possible traits grew and grew and also through lack of evidence on any substantial scale. There is some evidence that intelligence and physical energy are important in leadership and

Table 2.1: Conceptual perspectives on leadership

Conceptual approach	Definitions/models	Features
Personal qualities of the leader	Defined in terms of personality and behaviours of individual leaders	Individual behaviours and attitudes Personality traits Learned skills and capabilities Concerned with standards of personal effectiveness
Organisational positions	Defined in terms of formal organisational leadership roles, position, authority and/or professional status, for example, line management, expertise, reflected in both hierarchical and distributed or dispersed forms of leadership	Status and/or profession Organisational and personal authority Often associated with senior or supervisory roles Linked to organisational effectiveness
Leadership as social process	Defined in terms of social interaction with 'followers' with an emphasis on social influence attempts, communication, empathy for others, empowerment and coaching of others	Relational Influencing/motivational skills Effects on followers

these are influenced by genetics and early childhood experiences. A number of writers emphasise particular qualities such as integrity, self-confidence, self-awareness and resilience (Lord et al, 1986; Locke, 1991; Yukl, 2006), which may be partly innate and partly learned. But most modern leadership research suggests that leaders are not born but are largely made (and developed).

The literature from the mid-20th century focused on the behaviours, skills, mindsets and abilities of leaders, and here there is a large literature, which will be examined more fully in a later chapter (on the capabilities of leadership). For example, considerable research has been undertaken to try to identify the behaviours that distinguish effective from less effective leaders, such as behaviours showing concern for people and concern for the task (see, for example, Ohio State University studies by Fleishman et al, 1955) and getting the appropriate balance between these two dimensions. The work on transformational and transactional leadership falls under the behavioural approach to leadership (Burns, 1978; Bass, 1985), as does work on charismatic leadership (Bryman,

1992) and the more recent interest in mindsets (Ryde, 2007). Bennis and Thomas (2002) suggest that leaders are people with particular qualities or traits who are shaped by the formative experience of leadership. More recently, there has also been work on the dark side of leadership, which focuses on the traits and behaviours that can derail leaders or undermine effectiveness (Burke, 2006b).

Other work has considered the idea that individual leaders may vary their style according to the task and/or the context (for example, Fiedler, 1967; House and Dessler, 1974).

These approaches to leadership have been called leader-centric in that they focus on the characteristics of the leader. The role of individuals with their personal qualities in shaping events and circumstances at certain times is clear. The disadvantage of such approaches is that they can idealise particular individuals and assume that they have pre-eminent capacity and power, which ignores 'followers' and organisational and community constraints. This has been called the romance of leadership (Meindl and Ehrlich, 1987) in that the pre-eminence of the leader may be as much a social construction by 'followers' due to their own feelings and thoughts as due to the actual qualities of the leader.

In fact, Bryman (1992) argues that effective leadership by individuals is an interaction of the individual with their context. Sinclair (2005) argues that the lack of women in senior leadership positions is better explained by how society defines leadership than the qualities of women as leaders. Despite the limitations of taking a solely person-based perspective, however, Alimo-Metcalfe and Lawler (2001) note that a number of organisations are still taking a 'strong leader' approach to their leadership development programmes, with this focus on the individual and his/her personality. The 'strong leader' approach is also found in a number of policy documents in relation to the leadership of public organisations (Hartley and Allison, 2000) and this includes the health sector.

Leadership as position

Leadership can also be conceptualised in terms of organisational position or role. For example, in the NHS, this includes chief executives, medical directors, nurse managers and so on. A chief executive is in a position of authority, which may be a basis for leadership as well as management. Much of the leadership literature has conflated leadership with role, as it has drawn on research with the military or with business managers. Some commentators (for example, Rost, 1998) say that such formal positions give authority, and hence potentially the legitimacy to lead, but that the exercise of authority is not necessarily leadership. Leadership requires more than simply holding a particular office or role. Heifetz (1994) distinguishes between leadership with authority and leadership without (or beyond) authority, and formal and informal leadership. He argues that each may tackle leadership issues through different processes – for example, informal leaders may work through influence rather than through authority or direct control. Bryman (1992) notes that insufficient research has been directed to understanding informal leadership (for example from peers, or from outside the organisation).

As Hartley and Hinksman (2003) suggest, position within an organisation is one key indicator of leadership. A formal position within an organisation, such as chief executive or team leader or clinical consultant, brings with it the authority and legitimacy to lead others. In terms of social relationships, those in formal positions of authority are most likely to be regarded by staff as being in a leadership role as a result of the power and influence connected to the role they exercise in the working environment.

In healthcare organisations, leadership may be reinforced by the status or prestige of the formal role within the hierarchy. For example, the chief executive, director or chair of the board may be accorded legitimacy and even prestige because of their senior position, and, as a consequence of this position, they have the opportunity to exert greater influence than someone further down the pecking order. This is particularly relevant for complex healthcare systems where there are different types and sizes of organisational structures and cultures, including clinical teams, small clinical practices, multi-agency organisations, independent specialist providers and large hospitals.

However, leadership is clearly not solely about position, because there are many examples of ineffective leadership within particular roles – as well as many examples of leadership taking place outside or beyond the formal role.

Furthermore, leadership is not only found at the top of the organisation or in senior roles in teams. Writers have noted and commented on distributed or dispersed leadership in a variety of organisations including in health and in schools (Denis et al, 2001; Gronn, 2002; Spillane, 2005), for example, a team leader may operate with influence from a range of people in the team. Indeed discussion and debate about the efficacy of leadership in healthcare organisations is often concerned with questions about leadership across professional and managerial boundaries, both formal and informal, within single organisations and across organisational boundaries. We will explore this further in the Chapter 3 – here we note particularly the idea (concept) of leadership being based in organisational position, role or power.

The extent to which, for example, NHS chief executives are authoritative as leaders is complicated by their relationships with both politicians who set the policy context and clinicians on whose professional expertise healthcare delivery relies. The capacity for both these groups within and outside the organisation to affect the leadership of senior managers is significant. The expectations on chief executives to achieve organisational change, improvement and innovation are high, but charismatic 'celebrity' bosses who do achieve transformation by virtue of their position have been described as 'dangerous leaders' who may achieve much in the short term but leave their organisations destabilised (Buchanan, 2003).

Leadership as a social process

Leadership research in general has emphasised the importance of not just formal authority but also influence (it occurred in many of the definitions earlier). This involves thinking about leadership as a relationship and set of processes occurring between those trying to influence and those being influenced. Influence may occur at the team or group level, at the organisational level or at the societal level.

Influence may involve authority and/or formal power or it may involve mobilising and engaging others, for example through vision, passion or the clear articulation of goals. As this view of leadership is about processes, there is a need to also consider the relationships between 'leaders' and 'followers' – and also processes of mutual influence, because 'followers' may shape the kinds of approaches that leaders use (Collinson, 2006; Shamir et al, 2007).

Much of the work on leadership in healthcare has focused on leadership as a social process with the accent on how people in leadership positions transform organisations through influencing other people.

Acknowledging leadership as a social process suggests that effective leaders need to engage the hearts and minds of colleagues, staff and stakeholders to achieve leadership goals. This means taking care of relationships both internally and externally. Ferlie and Pettigrew (1996) have underlined the importance of external as well as internal relationships in a network-based approach to leadership that is increasingly important in healthcare. For example, Goodwin (1998) summarises the network of external relationships for a trust chief executive, showing the need to establish relationships including with

NHS providers, GPs, the private sector, local government, voluntary organisations, consumer groups, community groups, trade unions, local MPs and the media.

The social interaction aspects of leadership are also at the heart of another influential conceptual approach: adaptive leadership (Heifetz, 1994), which will be explored further in Chapter 5 on the challenges of leadership.

Studies of clinical leadership now recognise the importance of relationship management (for example, Millward and Bryan, 2005) and the need for emotional intelligence and coaching skills to achieve this (Henochowicz and Hetherington, 2006). Paying attention to the interrelational aspects of leadership is also reflected in the notion of 'communicative', 'democratic' or 'shared' leadership, which highlights the importance of discussion and deliberation as a means of organisational development to empower staff (Jackson, 2000; Eriksen, 2001). In their case study of nurse leaders in New Zealand for example, Kan and Parry (2004) acknowledge leadership as a social process, arguing that it contributes to a better understanding of the group dynamics between nurse leaders, nurses and other professional groups, and highlighting the importance of networking, coalition building and persuasion. Similarly McDonagh (2006) points to the importance of the governing board as a site for deliberative processes that provide organisational leadership.

As we have indicated earlier, leadership is multifaceted and can be conceptualised in a number of ways. Here, we have concentrated on three major strands or perspectives, about the person, the position and the process. Each has something to contribute to our understanding of leadership but each is deficient if applied in isolation on its own. Different writers emphasise these perspectives to different degrees and so it can be helpful to be aware of this in discussing and analysing leadership in healthcare.

Leadership or management?

It is not so long since everyone was arguing that 'management' was the answer to improving organisations, so why is there now a focus on leadership?

There are varied views about whether 'management' and 'leadership' are different or basically the same, as activities (not roles) within organisations. For example, Kotter (1990) argues that organisations need both leadership and management but that they are different: leadership is concerned with setting a direction for change, developing a vision for the future, while management consists of implementing those goals through planning, budgeting, staffing and so on. Others concur with this view (for example, Zaleznik, 1977; Bennis and Nanus, 1985). Kotter (1990) comments that most organisations are over-managed and under-led. Table 2.2 gives some commonly understood (though perhaps slightly caricatured) views of leadership activities compared with management activities, which some writers consider to be valid.

Table 2.2: Managers versus leaders

Managers	Leaders
Are transactional	Are transformative
Seek to operate and maintain current systems	Seek to challenge and change systems
Accept given objectives and meanings	Create new visions and meanings
Control and monitor	Empower
Trade on exchange relationships	Seek to inspire and transcend
Have a short-term focus	Have a long-term focus
Focus on detail and procedure	Focus on the strategic big picture

Source: Storey (2004)

However, there is an alternative view that is also strongly held. Yukl (2006) argues that defining leadership and management as distinct roles, processes or relationships may obscure more than it reveals: "Most scholars seem to agree that success as a manager or an administrator in modern organizations necessarily involves leading" (pp 6–7). Many studies of leadership have been based on managers in any case, so clearly some managers can be assumed also to be leaders (although being a manager does not per se make one a leader). Mintzberg (1973) described leadership as a key managerial role.

So managers are potentially leaders but they are not the only ones. Leadership is broader than management because it involves influence processes with a wide range of people, not just those who are in a relationship based on authority. It involves change but also can involve the routine; the transactional as well as the transformative.

The overlap, for many writers, between leadership and management is illustrated in Figure 2.2 on the next page

The debate about the relationship between management and leadership may in part be driven by the disciplinary interest of management theory, and the dominance of business schools in research and writing about leadership. Leadership analyses from different perspectives would pay as much attention to a variety of types of

Figure 2.2: The relationship between the activities of leadership and management

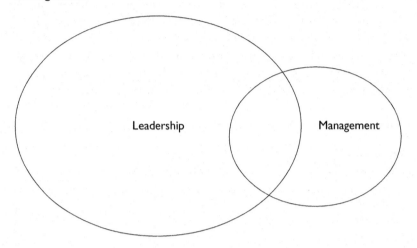

leadership in and around organisations. It is notable that the literature from healthcare specifically pays attention to medical leadership, clinical leadership and nurse leadership as well as to managerial leadership (for example, Berwick, 1994; Hackett and Spurgeon, 1998; Ham, 2003; Øvretveit, 2005a; Dickinson and Ham, 2008).

Anyone who influences others can be seen as a leader and therefore the leadership is not just the top managers or consultants in a hospital or surgery or Primary Care Trust. Nurses, occupational therapists, ward sisters and many others may at particular times and in particular contexts work in ways that exercise leadership. Clinical leadership and professional leadership are as important as managerial leadership in healthcare settings.

Leadership is multifaceted. Understanding leadership requires an understanding of the relationship between the behaviours of individuals in leadership positions and those they seek to influence.

Policy and practice implications:

- Too many studies fail to define what they mean by leadership. Creating an evidence base about leadership will be helped by clarity about how the term is used.
- How leadership is understood will have an impact on how and where we recognise (and accept) leadership. If leadership is seen as primarily about particular individuals with special accomplishments (heroic individuals), then there may be under-recognition of the contributions that others in the team or unit can make.
- If leadership is understood as primarily about position in the organisation then the focus on leadership will be primarily on the upper echelons of the organisation and the opportunity to cultivate and practise distributed leadership may be impaired.
- If the concept of leadership is pictured primarily in terms of social processes of influence and mobilisation, then attention will need to be paid to how the leader understands, interacts with and engages with the group. Leadership through influence requires the cultivation of interpersonal skills and emotional intelligence, among other things.
- 'Followers' have a responsibility to think about how they can influence and support, if appropriate, the formal leader in the group's tasks.
- In practice, leadership may have elements of all three of the concepts of person, position and process in various combinations.
- The concept of leadership also shapes how leadership development is viewed. A focus on the individual will mean particular emphasis on selecting and developing individuals. A focus on organisational position may mean that only particular positions in the organisation are given certain types of training and development in leadership skills. A focus on social processes will mean some development emphasis on working in groups and teams.
- 'Talent spotting' for people with leadership potential, for example, fast-track trainees, clinical staff shifting into managerial roles and so on, will be affected by the leadership concept used.
- Confusion about leadership can sometimes be avoided by paying attention to how people understand and use the term leadership.

CHAPTER 3

Characteristics of leadership

In this chapter:

We examine different types of leadership, rather than assuming that there is a generic form of leadership. The chapter examines those aspects of leadership that provide the bases of influence. This is about exploring the roles and resources of different types of leadership. The chapter makes distinctions between formal and informal leadership, arguing that each has particular sources of power and influence, as well as advantages and disadvantages. The chapter then examines direct (local) and indirect (distant) leadership, clinical and non-clinical leadership, and political and managerial leadership on the same basis, before looking at individual and shared/distributed leadership. The different roles provide different bases of authority and of legitimacy. The chapter also examines the sources of power and influence.

In examining the characteristics of leadership, we turn to the next segment in the leadership framework, shown in Figure 3.1.

Figure 3.1: The characteristics of leadership

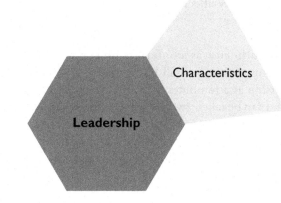

Who are the leaders in healthcare?

If leadership is thought of as the process of influencing people in the formulation or pursuit of goals, then potentially everyone working in healthcare can be a leader at some time, for some purposes. On the other hand, there are differences between the context, power base, purposes and practice of leadership between, say, a hospital chief executive and a ward sister, or a medical director and a Department of Health policy advisor. Some leadership in healthcare is also practised outside the formal healthcare organisation, for example, by patient groups, by MPs and by local government councillors involved in health scrutiny. Should they all be treated as the same, in terms of their leadership? Or, should we consider how their roles and their resources have an impact on the kinds of leadership that can be exercised, and on what basis? This chapter is concerned with defining some of the characteristics of varied types of leadership in order to understand more about how they influence other people, groups and goals. This takes us into a consideration of the roles of leaders and the resources they have available to them (sources of power and influence) in both organisational and network settings in healthcare.

Formal and informal leadership

The work of the Harvard academic Ron Heifetz (1994) is useful in drawing the distinction between formal and informal leadership. Heifetz argues that the basis of authority provides different opportunities for and constraints on exercising leadership. He makes a crucial distinction between leadership *with* authority and leadership *without* authority. He argues that leadership research has made insufficient distinction between these, yet they affect the strategies of leading that are open to the person or group:

> I define authority as conferred power to perform a service. This definition will be useful to the practitioner of leadership as a reminder of two facts: First, authority is given and can be taken away. Second, authority is conferred as part of an exchange. Failure to meet the terms of the exchange means the risk of losing one's authority: it can be taken back or given to another who promises to fulfill the bargain. (1994, p 57)

Leadership with authority can also be called positional power (power that derives from a position of authority). The conferring of power, in the quotation earlier, emphasises that formal authority is given by other people, whether this occurs through election or appointment. Formal authority is an important source of leadership in healthcare (for example, the authority that is accepted and indeed expected from those in senior positions, whether clinical or managerial). Heifetz notes that not all authority relationships are based on a conscious conferring of power because sometimes people defer to those in authority out of habitual deference and do not realise the power they have to withhold legitimacy from the person claiming authority: "in our organizations and our politics, we look generally to our authorities for direction, protection and order" (Heifetz, 1994, p 69).

This emphasises that there is an interdependent relationship between those in authority and those who accept (or resist or resent) authority. Authority is important in the analysis of leadership because the personal qualities of the individual are not the whole story; leadership may be a combination of personal qualities, authority and the relationship(s) with the people who are being led or influenced.

Leadership without authority, also called informal leadership, has a different base and therefore a different set of activities associated with it. These are individuals and groups who lead societies, communities, groups or particular issues (either inside or outside the organisation) and influence others without formal authorisation, for example, a campaigning group or an expert whose views people regard seriously, even though that person is not in a formal position of authority.

A leader acting without authority may be less constrained by the roles and rules, and by the expectations of others (that is, those who confer the authority) but there are also risks. Informal leaders, says Heifetz, have two advantages. First, they have more latitude for creative deviance; for example, they can dramatise for effect, or they can focus on a single issue, or they can press for action without having to look at the larger picture or balance competing priorities. They can campaign on issues with energy. Second, they may have close contact with the detailed experiences of some of the stakeholders and therefore have crucial information about the front-line that can be much harder for those in authority positions to gain. For example, think of a health campaigner compared with an NHS chief executive, to get a sense of the different roles they have and the sources of leadership influence that they use and to which they have access.

The strategies of informal leaders may be "both more bold and subtle" (Heifetz, 1994, p 207) than those of leaders with formal authority. Informal leaders can spark debate but may find it harder than formal leaders to orchestrate the ensuing discussion between stakeholders. They have depth of experience on the front-line but may be less aware of other wider aspects of the problem; they may get attacked for their views but have fewer resources to deflect the heat. They also have to think hard about how, and when and if, to challenge established authority because it is all too easy to be deflected into challenging the authority figure at the expense of achieving goals. An informal leader also has to decide when to bypass authority and look for other ways to achieve outcomes (Hartley and Fletcher, 2008).

There are all kinds of informal leaders in healthcare, whether these are influential clinicians, whose views are highly regarded, or front-line staff who are particularly persuasive with their peers, patients and others. There are also informal leaders outside the formal health structures, such as patient groups advocating particular types or levels of care, or journalists whose articles shape public opinion. In different ways, each of these can shape perceptions of and commitment to goals and outcomes in health, whether locally or nationally.

Some research has pointed to the importance of a particular category of informal leaders within healthcare, namely 'opinion leaders'. For example, Locock and colleagues (2001) evaluated the literature on evidence-based practice and found a strong role for opinion leaders. Their influence was based less on their formal role and more on their international research reputation, their commanding of respect from others and their understanding of the realities of clinical practice. Locock et al found two types of opinion leader – those who were experts in their field, and those who were well regarded by their peers (not necessarily exclusive categories). They also found that these informal roles served different purposes at different stages of the implementation of evidence-based practice. At the early stage, the expert can have more influence, but in the implementation stage, the peer may have more influence.

Strong opinion leaders may lead in resisting change being proposed by others. Øvretveit (2005b), in a review of the healthcare literature on leading quality and safety improvements, found that identifying and influencing the opinion leaders among doctors was an important means of influencing improvements in healthcare quality and safety.

Direct and indirect leadership

A number of writers make a distinction between direct (or 'near' or 'local' leadership) and indirect (or 'distant') leadership (Hunt, 1991;

Yammarino, 1994; Alimo-Metcalfe and Alban-Metcalfe, 2002; Millward and Bryan, 2005; Yukl, 2006).

Direct face-to-face leadership occurs where the size of the group allows frequent, interpersonal contact and it often occurs at the front-line. This is where others in the team or group are used to seeing the leader daily or regularly in face-to-face working. Direct leaders are able to get to know those they work with and influence them on an interpersonal basis. They are likely to know all the members of the group that they are leading. They are able to develop members of their group through one-to-one relationships and they are close enough to see quite quickly when things are going well or badly. They have an important role in empowering nursing staff (Laschinger et al, 1999). Yukl (2006) notes that most theories of leadership are based on the assumption that leaders are able to directly influence those they work with (because the majority of studies have been conducted on managers and their immediate subordinates). In the context of healthcare, one can think of direct leadership as being embodied in the ward sister, or the consultant who is head of an operating team, or the leader of a cancer collaborative.

By contrast, indirect leadership is exercised where the leader has an influence on others through the chain of command in the organisation or through forms of positional influence, but where the relationship is too distant to be based on personal interaction. The leadership of a Secretary of State for Health or a chief executive is of this type. In such leadership, influence is not on an interpersonal basis but takes place, for instance, through mass communication (for example, newsletters, videos, large meetings, mass media) and also through policies and procedures. It is not possible for indirect leaders to influence the group or organisation through direct relationships and so part of their approach may be to try to create and communicate the overall goals, values and behaviours that are expected from organisational members. This is one of the reasons why indirect leaders are concerned to formulate a compelling vision and clear goals for the organisation, to shape the organisational climate and to communicate the compelling vision. Effective indirect leaders are also aware of the value of symbolic acts in communicating culture or values (Hatch, 1997; Schein, 2004). When a chief executive spends time 'on the shop floor' or working for a short period alongside front-line staff, they get a stronger sense of the front-line tasks and challenges, and their presence and actions also communicate symbolically the importance of a user focus.

Some indirect health leaders may not work inside the organisation at all, but, for example, in central government or in one of the more influential think-tanks. Policy-makers such as ministers or policy advisors in the Department of Health aim to be significant healthcare leaders, although they will meet only a fraction of those whose work they are trying to influence.

Direct and indirect leadership are not mutually exclusive. For example, a hospital chief executive will be a direct leader in relation to his/her own management team, but will be an indirect leader for the hospital staff overall, some of whom may rarely or never see the chief executive, but their work will be shaped by his/her actions.

The distinction between direct and indirect leadership is valuable for considering how influence takes place and the scale and scope of the context. What works in a face-to-face daily situation may not work at all in a situation of indirect leadership (and vice versa).

Clinical and non-clinical leadership

Clinical leadership (whether by doctors, nurses or other medical professions) has both a different purpose ('challenge' in the language of this book) and a different influence base compared with non-clinical leadership. It has been suggested that the focus of clinical leadership is "about facilitating evidence-based practice and improved patient outcomes through local care" (Millward and Bryan, 2005, p 15). On the other hand, empire-building and self-protection is also sometimes evident. The influence base for clinical leadership, especially medical leadership, has two main sources. It is partly collective (the power and influence that comes through professional associations such as Royal Colleges, or the Royal Societies of each profession), and partly based in individual clinical expertise (Ferlie and Pettigrew, 1996; Goodwin, 2000; Millward and Bryan, 2005; Souba and Day, 2006). The professional power base of doctors in particular sometimes makes collaboration between managerial and clinical leadership quite difficult (Millward and Bryan, 2005; Dickinson and Ham, 2008). It creates particular dilemmas for clinical managers, who lead on the boundaries between clinical and managerial work (Marnoch et al, 2000; Sheaff et al, 2003).

We found less written about clinical leadership by doctors than about nurse leadership (although see Willcocks, 2005; Clark et al, 2008; Dickinson and Ham, 2008; Ham, 2008). A recent review of the literature on leadership by doctors (Dickinson and Ham, 2008) found that doctors play key leadership roles, although these roles require greater attention, and that dispersed and collective leadership among doctors is important and under-researched. The review also noted a continuing influence of informal leaders and networks operating alongside formal structures.

There is a larger literature about nurse leadership, mainly of direct leadership and mainly concerned with the impact of leadership rather than its sources of authority and legitimacy. Understanding effective clinical-managerial leadership relationships remains an important issue (for example, Weiner et al, 1997; Dickinson and Ham, 2008).

The need to understand clinical leadership across a variety of health professions is given added impetus by the Darzi report (DH, 2008), which sets out the importance of clinical leadership for the UK health service, its contribution to clinical practice, to working in partnerships (in health teams and with partners outside the health service such as social care) and to leading the organisation in research, education and service delivery.

Political and organisational leadership

Healthcare across the world attracts considerable attention from national and local elected politicians (Goodwin, 2000, 2006; Ferlie and Shortell, 2001), and the NHS in the UK and the healthcare system in the US are hotly contested by their publics as well. Political leadership is relevant to healthcare particularly where politicians set policy and financial resource allocations for the healthcare organisations, and comment on the successes and failures of healthcare. They may become involved in controversial decisions by health organisations, for example, over mergers or closures of hospitals, or over drugs policy or patient safety policy. In addition, politicians are involved at the local level through the scrutiny of local policies and practices, for example, the health overview and scrutiny body of the local authority in the area of a hospital or Primary Care Trust (PCT) (see, for example, Coleman and Glendinning, 2004). In the UK, the scope for discretion at local level by clinicians and managers is constrained by the political leadership exercised both in Parliament and through the Department of Health, by the politics and budgets of Strategic Health Authorities and PCTs and in terms of local public opinion by local government politicians. Political leadership differs from organisational leadership in its basis of authority. Politicians are elected not appointed and they have a responsibility to make decisions on behalf of all the various stakeholders who elected them and with regard for the well-being of future generations (Morrell and Hartley, 2006; Hartley, 2010b). The basis of power for politicians lies in the ballot box, in their support from the electorate and from their colleagues in their political party (or coalition), whether at local or national level. As a consequence they have to address complex goals that are sometimes in tension (Leach et al, 2005; Simpson, 2008). In addition, those in health governance roles, such as board members, have to interact with the political world, and therefore political awareness, in terms of understanding the institutions and processes of government, and the needs of diverse stakeholders can be important (Hartley and Fletcher, 2008).

Individual and shared/distributed leadership

Some leadership is exercised by individuals, often because they are in a role of formal authority, exerting leadership through the organisational hierarchy:

> In academic medicine, we tend to think of leadership as being about a person in charge who wields power and stands apart. The word 'leader' may bring to mind vivid images: the gifted surgeon who pioneers a new procedure; the brilliant researcher who advances our understanding of a disease.... By and large, our view of leadership tends to centre around visible individuals and their talents, contributions and achievements. This view of leadership is not wrong, but it is no longer adequate. (Souba, 2004, p 177)

It is increasingly recognised that it is becoming more and more difficult for a single person to accomplish the work of leadership, because of the pace and volatility of change in the external environment, whether in the private or public sectors. So leaders have to understand, lead, shape, manage and react to change with higher levels of uncertainty and risk than in the past (Marion and Uhl-Bien, 2001; Benington and Hartley, 2009). Knowledge needs to be shared across teams and across organisations in order to achieve quality outcomes. And if new ways of working are to be implemented effectively, then some leadership tasks may need to be shared. For example, in PCTs the collaborative leadership roles and relationships between the trust chair, chief executive and Professional Executive Committee chair/clinical lead is increasingly important. Other examples include cancer collaboratives, the productive ward and inter-organisational partnership working, which all require some degree of shared leadership. Shared leadership is particularly relevant to working in partnerships inside and outside the organisation and in inter-organisational networks (Hartley and Allison, 2000; Gronn, 2002; Jackson and Parry, 2008).

It has been noted that shared leadership is more complicated and time-consuming than individual leadership (Burke, 2006a) and for these reasons it is most effectively deployed where the tasks:

- are highly interdependent
- are highly complex
- require creativity.

These are the situations where adaptive leadership (Heifetz, 1994) often comes into play, which involves engaging others in recognising that the problems are complex, have no technical answer and that the group members themselves, among others, have a role to play in solving them. Such conditions are often present in healthcare and Ferlie and Shortell (2001) argue that the idea of a single charismatic health leader needs to be replaced with an emphasis on shared and distributed leadership across teams and networks for effective clinical care and organisational change.

In some situations, there may be both individual leadership (through vertical lines of authority) combined with shared leadership, as, for example, in teams that have an acknowledged head or formal leader in terms of accountability and responsibility but where a number of members in the team may contribute to the work of leadership.

In situations of organisational ambiguity and major change, there may need to be a 'leadership constellation' whereby the leadership role passes, informally or at different phases, between different individuals and groups, with differing bases of expertise and legitimacy at different times. This was found in health restructuring in Canada (Denis et al, 2001). This may happen in various complex change situations, for example, in mergers, reconfigurations and restructurings.

A slightly different strand of the shared leadership approach is that of 'distributed leadership'. This signals a shift from heroic individual leaders towards collective or distributed leadership (Parry and Bryman, 2006). This is part of the approach of seeing leadership as "leading others to lead themselves" (Sims and Lorenzi, cited in Parry and Bryman, 2006, p 296; see also Kouzes and Posner, 1995). It is captured in the notion of transformational leadership, which, among other things, argues that leadership includes strengthening the capacity of others to be empowered and to lead themselves. It has been argued that the greatest leadership challenge for leaders is to enable others to act and to build leadership capacity in the organisation (Kouzes and Posner, 1995; Fullan, 2001).

The notion of distributed leadership brings us close to considering leadership as a quality of the whole organisation, network or system. Dispersed or distributed leadership is based on the idea that leadership can be exercised at different levels of an organisation and is not just the preserve of senior executives. Dispersed leadership challenges the traditional assumptions that leaders are superior to their followers (Ray et al, 2004). When leadership skills and responsibilities are decentralised, or shared across different elements of a task (Denis et al, 2001), there is a new focus on sharing knowledge and power as well as dispersing leadership. Distributed leadership acknowledges that the role of senior leaders is sometimes less to lead from the front than to enable others to lead. In so doing, the dependence (or sometimes over-dependence) of followers on formal leadership figures decreases and the whole group may become more empowered (Buchanan, 2003).

In healthcare organisations, particularly when innovation and change for improvement is required, dispersed leadership by change agents throughout the organisation may be particularly valuable. Denis et al (1996, 2001) demonstrate this in their work in Canadian hospitals at a time of strategic change, while Neath (2007) reports on the significance of devolved leadership for Strategic Health Authorities in a study of the National Booking Programme from 1998 to 2003 in the UK. Williams (2004a) argues for the importance of recognising the multilayered nature of leadership throughout the organisation in implementing change through information technology in health, while Jackson and Parry (2008) note that the new information technologies and systems are creating new opportunities and challenges in relation to distributed leadership. Dopson et al (2005) have also highlighted the role of 'opinion leaders' at all levels of the organisation in encouraging or blocking healthcare reform, suggesting that their impact will be affected by their profile (for example, as professional expert) and location within the organisation.

Leading clinical teams can be described as a form of distributed leadership, since it requires management of a range of relationships between professionals, managers and service users, particularly when working in a multidisciplinary or multi-agency context (Millward and Bryan, 2005). Such forms of dispersed leadership rely on the professional and personal authority of leaders and their skills in coalition-building and inter-organisational networking, not just their location in the hierarchy of the organisation. Studies of nurse leaders also reinforce the importance of organisations recognising and supporting informal as well as formal leadership roles. Those in dispersed medical or nurse leadership roles will need to be recognised and supported as transformational leaders in order to effect sustainable organisational change and improvement (Millward and Bryan, 2005). Others acknowledge that there is an interplay between dispersed leadership and location in the formal hierarchy and that clinical staff leaders have unequal access to sources of power (Manojilovich, 2005).

Roles and sources of influence in organisational and network settings

This review of the characteristics of leadership indicates the range of roles and resources (authority, expertise, near or distant influence and so on) that have an impact on the ways in which leadership is exercised in organisational and societal settings. Each may shape the goals, the processes and the outcomes of healthcare, and there may be tensions between different leadership roles.

However, most of the leadership literature does not make clear what aspects of leadership are being studied. For example, is the focus on direct or indirect leadership? Is it concerned with leadership based on formal authority or on informal leadership? (Most research has taken place within organisational settings, resulting in the conflation of leadership with formal authority.) On what basis is leadership being exercised? The types of influence, the behaviours, the sources of legitimacy and the types of relationships that can be established will vary according to the basis of leadership.

Leadership varies in its scope (direct or indirect), in its role (formal or informal authority; political, managerial or professional; clinical or non-clinical) and in the sources of power and influence that can be used.

If leadership is partly an influence process within a group or between groups of people, then leadership is not only about the behaviours of the leader but about the willingness or ability of others to accept or resist influence. Yukl (2006) summarises the research evidence on different types of power, using and extending the conceptualisation of sources of power from French and Raven (1959). Yukl uses this work to distinguish between position power (derived from the person's position in the organisation) and personal power (derived from attributes of the person and their relationship with those being influenced). A summary is shown in Table 3.1.

Power is not a substance but a relationship. In common language we often talk about someone 'having power' but in fact they only have power to the extent that this is accepted by those who are being influenced. For example, legitimate power (formal authority) is a source of influence upon those who accept the explicit norms (for example,

Table 3.1: Different bases of power

Positional power	Personal power
• Legitimate power (formal authority) • Reward power (power to provide rewards) • Coercive power (power to provide punishments or sanctions) • Information power (access to and control over information) • Ecological power (control over the physical environment, technology, organisation of work and organisational culture)	• Referent power (desire of others to please the leader due to strong feelings of affection, admiration or loyalty. Charisma is one type of referent power) • Expert power (task-relevant knowledge and skill)

Source: Adapted from Yukl (2006)

the results of a vote or an appointment process), who are loyal to the organisation and who agree with the organisational goals and values, or who have internalised values about accepting authority. Expert power operates where others recognise the person as having expertise, which does not derive from qualifications alone. Thus, power is a social process that depends on the quality of the interaction between both the leader and the people being influenced.

Positional power and personal power interact in complex ways and it is sometimes hard to distinguish their interrelationship in any particular situation. The analysis of sources of power helps to tease out the different types of influence that derive from different roles and relationships. This helps also to explain why direct leadership may operate differently from indirect leadership, and why clinical leadership has different characteristics from non-clinical leadership. It is possible to use Table 3.1 to analyse the sources of influence for many different types of leader.

Policy and practice implications:

- Much mainstream writing on leadership has assumed a uniformity of leadership – as though it is simply a universal process of influencing others and that there is 'one best approach' to leadership. But the consideration of leadership characteristics in this chapter shows that the roles and the resources (for example, authority, information, reputation, resources, expertise) can vary enormously. This explains why there are different types of leadership in and around healthcare organisations. It also explains why leadership cannot be considered solely from the point of view of individuals.

- This analysis also shows that leadership does not operate only at the top of the organisation (for example, in the board or in the senior teams) but can be distributed across the whole organisation, or spread across inter-organisational networks.

- Some leaders hold formal authority and are enabled to act with legitimacy on behalf of the organisation. But it is worth remembering that authority is conferred and accepted by others, so authority has to be used in ways that meet the approval of those who have conferred the authority.

- Informal leadership is also prevalent in and around many public services, including healthcare. Opinion leaders inside the organisation and campaigning groups outside the organisation are likely to be influential leaders but without formal authority. In thinking about leadership, it is worth taking account of who are the informal as well as the formal leaders who can have an impact on health outcomes.

- Clinical leadership is an increasingly important element of healthcare, where such leaders may be sources of influence directly as practitioners influencing others in their teams or departments, and may also be contributing to the wider management of the healthcare organisation. The sources of clinical leadership lie partly in expertise but effective leadership also involves being able to see the wider strategic view about healthcare delivery and organisation.

- Elected politicians are sometimes seen as an encumbrance to the efficient operations of healthcare but this view does not take into account their sources of legitimacy, their mandate or their goals to be achieved on behalf of the wider population, either locally or nationally.

- Leadership approaches will depend on whether the leader is a direct or an indirect leader. Much of the literature ignores this distinction but the sources of influence can be quite different. Indirect leadership requires influence through symbolic acts and through shaping the organisational goals, policies and practices.

- Shared, distributed or dispersed leadership is increasingly common and is particularly valuable for tasks that are complex, knowledge-intensive and where the outcomes are uncertain. Shared leadership requires a different set of skills from individual leadership.

- Shared leadership will become particularly important to understand the more that community enterprise organisations are encouraged to provide healthcare.
- There are varied sources of power in leadership. The distinction between positional power (power derived from a formal position of authority) and personal power is useful in analysing the sources of influence that both formal and informal leaders may use.
- There is not 'one best way' to be a leader – the opportunities to influence will partly depend on the power resources available from the individual, the organisation and the networks they are embedded in.

CHAPTER 4

The contexts of leadership

In this chapter:

What is 'context' and why is it important for leadership? This chapter examines the interactions between context and leadership, in terms of three layers: the public policy context of healthcare; the local strategic context (including working in partnerships); and the internal, organisational context. Context is relevant for leaders in several ways. It provides the constraints on and opportunities for action, and so a key skill for leaders is being able to 'read' the context. They also may shape the context in some situations and articulate and make sense of the context for other people.

An important strand of thinking in leadership studies is the relationship between what leaders do and the context in which they do it. First, how does leadership vary according to different contexts? Second, how can and do leaders shape the context in which they operate?

It is widely agreed that leadership is related to, or contingent on, context and that a key prerequisite of effective leadership is the ability

Figure 4.1: The contexts of leadership

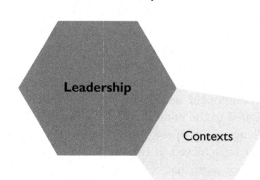

to understand that context. Theorists have looked at this from a number of perspectives, exploring both the influence of contextual factors on leadership, and the influence of leadership in shaping context. However, there is much less work than might be expected on this crucial set of interactions between leadership and context. Porter and McLaughlin (2006) review the theoretical and empirical knowledge about leadership and the organisational context (across all types of organisation) and conclude that there is little research that takes context into account as an analytical factor, rather than simply as part of the description of the location of a particular leadership case or situation. They argue for much more rigorous and systematic attention to understanding the impact of context on leadership and vice versa (see also Osborn et al, 2002). Grint (2000) thinks this issue of context is so important that he classifies theories about leadership according to the degree to which they pay attention to, or ignore, context as an aspect of leadership.

Goodwin (2006), writing about healthcare, observes that research has tended to focus on leadership as a determinant in shaping context, rather than vice versa – on political, economic, social and organisational context as determinants of leadership choices and styles.

Early work on leadership was influential in understanding how leadership varied by context, and the extent to which leadership was effective in its matching of leadership style to context (Fiedler, 1967; House and Dessler, 1974). Fiedler's work suggested that different leadership styles are more effective depending upon the level of control that a leader has in a situation. A leader with a 'task-orientation' can be most effective in circumstances of extremely high or low situational control, while a leader with a 'people-orientation' would be most effective in circumstances of moderate situational control. In other words, the leader should modify their style according to how much control they have over the situation they and the group are in.

This suggests that one key leadership skill is the ability to read different contexts and respond appropriately (Hartley et al, 2007; Hartley and Fletcher, 2008). Situational analysis by the leader or leadership team/ group is a key component in ensuring that the leadership strategy and style are aligned to the context. (This includes the nature of the leadership challenge, or purpose, which is covered in Chapter 5.) Alignment might be achieved in two ways. The first is by selecting particular leaders for particular contexts (for example, in Chapter 5 we examine how different leadership styles are useful in early stages compared with late stages of merger in healthcare). The second way is to encourage a leader to learn to be versatile, that is to adapt their style to the particular context. Different situations demand different leadership approaches, and a leader who can adapt to changing contextual factors is more likely to be regarded as competent (and therefore effective) than one who has a rigid, inflexible approach (Buchanan, 2003).

Reading the context includes being able to take an overview of the external and internal conditions and opportunities, and also being able to move between "the balcony and the battlefield" (Benington and Turbitt, 2007, p 384). This involves the ability to link the strategic big picture with the operational detail. Part of the skill lies in being able to sense the 'soft' points in the political, organisational or partnership context where the leader's priorities can be taken forward without provoking stubborn opposition (Leach et al, 2005).

Contingent or situational leadership perspectives acknowledge that leadership is carried out in a variety of dynamic situations with numerous contextual variables to take into account. In helping us to understand and explain effective leadership, theories which suggest that leadership is contingent on context are therefore only helpful up to a point. Yukl (2006) for example, suggests that "contingency theories do not provide sufficient guidance in the form of general principles to help managers recognize the underlying leadership requirements and choices in the myriad of fragmented activities and problems confronting them" (p 240).

Grint (2005b) goes a step further in discussing the interaction between leadership and context to argue that effective leaders not only shape the softer elements of context but also work to constitute the context. This 'constitutive' approach to leadership argues that leaders have a key role in making sense of the context and defining reality for those they are trying to influence. So, how they define a situation and frame it for others is a key element of leadership (see also Hartley, 2002a; Leach et al, 2005). We explore this 'sense-making' aspect of leadership as a crucial challenge in more detail in Chapter 5. Its relationship to the context is important.

Turning to the healthcare literature specifically, we found little on the impact of context on leadership. Reviews of the relationship between context and leadership hardly touched on the healthcare field (Porter and McLaughlin, 2006). However, the idea that the interaction of leaders with their organisational and external context is a critical element in achieving effective change and improvement is increasingly recognised.

Layers of context

We suggest that leadership in healthcare can be thought of as being situated within three 'layers of context'. Of course, the boundaries between the layers are blurred, and some aspects of context may be evident at more than one layer. We outline this mapping of context in Table 4.1.

Table 4.1: Layers of context in healthcare

Context	Focus
National political and public policy context	External political and policy environment
Regional and local context	Intermediate NHS 'system' at the level of the regional/local health economy
Internal organisational context	Internal organisational structure, culture, history, size, geography and resources

Layers of context are likely to be dynamic and changing. Leadership within healthcare organisations does not operate within a static context but rather needs to take account of fluctuations in public policy, political change and the organisation's performance level (and capacity for improvement).

Many writers on change management have argued that environmental or contextual volatility is a key factor to be taken into account in leading successful organisations, acknowledging that the structures and practices appropriate in stable conditions are not always fit for purpose in more unpredictable times (Dunphy and Stace, 1993; Greenwood and Hinings, 1996; Scott, 2001).

Whole-systems thinking is helpful to understand how these layers of context are part of an interconnected system of complex networks rather than mechanical and linear cause-and-effect relationships. Iles and Sutherland (2001) highlight the key points of understanding a complex and open system as:

- being made up of related and interdependent parts so that any system must be viewed as a whole;
- a system that should not be considered in isolation from its environment;
- being in equilibrium, which will only change if some type of energy is applied;
- comprising different players who will have different views of the system function and purpose.

In addition, they note that human activity systems are characterised by frequently multiple and often conflicting objectives.

It is helpful to take a systems view of the context of healthcare, with its myriad influences on any particular healthcare organisation and thus on the leadership in and of that organisation. Leadership theory is increasingly taking account of whole-systems thinking and analysis (for example, Wheatley, 1992; Marion and Uhl-Bien, 2001; Benington and Hartley, 2009; Uhl-Bien and Marion, 2009).

The national public policy context

National healthcare systems can be said to be 'context heavy'. They are necessarily affected by political, economic and social factors from the wider society. Chapter 1 outlined some of the pressures on health organisations and health economies of changes in health needs, public expectations, financial provision and so on. For example, increased consumer expectations alongside medical-technological advances and an ageing population have put increasing pressure on scarce resources for healthcare. The importance of preventative strategies and the promotion of health rather than expanding remedial responses to sickness is prompting new ways of thinking about healthcare provision in the UK. Political imperatives to meet increased demand and also achieve value for money and promote efficiencies have led to measures to foster innovation and improvement in healthcare (for example, to improve quality, safety, speed and efficiency in the provision of services). The role of central government in driving change through legislation, statutory guidance, financial control and performance measurement is a dominant contextual factor.

In England, *The NHS Plan* (DH, 2000) set the framework for modernising the NHS over a 10-year period and this has been followed up with the Darzi review and report (DH, 2008). These documents provide an ambitious national strategy, with a vision for healthcare designed around the needs of patients and with increased local responsibility and accountability for meeting nationally set quality and performance standards. The leadership challenge is explicitly to transform services in order to improve, and create step-change through innovation. The financial crisis and predictions of reduced public expenditure from 2011 onwards create further challenges to 'do more with less' while maintaining quality and safety.

Leaders in healthcare thus have to operate within a context and a system in almost constant flux, including:

- the creation of independent Foundation Trust hospitals with governors elected from the hospital membership;

- the drive to increase capacity within healthcare services through the voluntary sector, independent service providers and community enterprises;
- the reconfiguration of Primary Care Trusts (PCTs), resulting in a smaller number of PCTs generally aligned to local authority boundaries;
- the local commissioning of services by PCTs and GPs;
- the introduction of increased patient choice of services, for example, the 'choose and book' appointments system;
- a stringent regime of national performance targets, with central government intervention for underperforming organisations;
- a greater emphasis on innovation and continuous improvement in healthcare and in healthcare management;
- greater local accountability to councillors of the local authority through new health overview and scrutiny committees;
- increasing financial pressures after an extended period of growth in healthcare funding.

All these factors result, or will result, in a significantly changed context for leadership in healthcare. Understanding where and how leadership operates within such a complex context is an important prerequisite for success. In his study of NHS chief executives, Blackler (2006) records the pressures that health service chief executives were subject to as "conduits for the policies of the centre" (p 5) rather than providing the scope to help lead the reform of the NHS. He reports NHS chief executives "having to function in an increasingly rigid hierarchy in which there was a lot of fear", suggesting that they "needed to ignore uncertainties, were being forced to impose centrally determined priorities on their staff and were being held personally responsible for performance outcomes". His conclusion that "the popular image of empowered, proactive leaders has little relevance to the work of the NHS chief executive" (p 15) underlines the central role of national government in shaping the context in which chief executives exercise leadership.

Goodwin (2000) acknowledges the impact of the wider political environment on leaders in the NHS, pointing out the importance of external relationships and inter-organisational networking in helping to counterbalance local priorities against the "backcloth of national, government determined aims for public services" (p 56) and suggesting that future leaders "will have to be dependent not only upon establishing a successful partnership with politicians and professionals but also achieving greater inter-organisational collaboration by transcending traditional organizational boundaries" (p 58).

These national policies and their local impacts increase the challenge facing leadership to achieve sustainable and substantial change. This is a significant element of the context for leadership in healthcare. The *Next stage review* (DH, 2008) acknowledges the problems that have been engendered in earlier stages of recent restructurings and other changes in the NHS system, and aims to address this, in part by strengthening clinical and non-clinical leadership.

The regional and local context

A further layer of context is that of the regional or local healthcare system. 'Reading the context' at this level involves two key elements. The first is how to interpret the complex interrelationships at the regional/local level, and the second is how to lead effectively in this context.

Public policy has been in almost continuous system change over recent years with the introduction of different forms of organisational governance, merged organisations and an increased emphasis on interdisciplinary and inter-organisational service delivery. Systems thinking is helpful in understanding how to lead in this context of complex networks of organisations interrelating, collaborating and competing to provide healthcare. There is increasing interest in how a systems approach may be helpful in understanding the NHS and its network of other private, public and voluntary sector providers of health and social care (Iles and Sutherland, 2001). A systems approach for healthcare involves:

- an awareness of the multifactoral issues involved in healthcare, which mean that complex health and social problems lie beyond the ability of any one practitioner, team or agency to address;
- interest in designing, planning and managing organisations as dynamic, interdependent systems committed to providing 'seamless care' for patients;
- recognition of the need to develop shared values, purposes and practices within and between organisations;
- use of large group interventions to bring together the perspectives of a wide range of stakeholders across the whole healthcare system.

Leadership frameworks need to take account of the increases in the interrelationships between organisations, through networking, joint ventures and strategic alliances, and the greater impacts that stakeholders such as lobby and campaigning groups may have on organisations in the private, public and voluntary sectors (Hartley and Fletcher, 2008). Selznick (1957, p 23) argued that "the theory of leadership is dependent on the theory of organization". This means that as theories of organisations change, then theories of leadership need to change as well. Leadership that is able to influence not only colleagues and subordinates, but also a range of stakeholders and networks in the private, public and voluntary sectors is becoming increasingly important.

A number of commentators have noted the increasing use of inter-professional and inter-organisational networks and partnerships in the public service sector for the achievement of service outcomes (Benington, 2000, 2001; Stoker, 2006). However, as Goodwin (2006) notes, while the value of networks in healthcare is discussed, the amount of research is actually very low. Some discussion is in adulatory terms, but Benington (2001) has argued that while networks and partnerships have the advantages of flexibility and adaptability, they also have disadvantages in terms of 'steering' and accountability. Others have noted that as well as there being 'collaborative advantage' there can also be collaborative disadvantage (Huxham and Vangen, 2000).

The analysis of networks suggests that this is an important aspect of healthcare leadership, but that there is still insufficient research both on the processes and outcomes of networks, let alone the implications for leadership and leadership skills.

The context at this intermediate regional and local level is one of interrelationships between a complex network of commissioners, providers, regulators, opinion-formers and advocacy groups. The network may also include those organisations whose activities have an impact on public health and on community healthcare, such as the local authority, the police and the voluntary sector. There is a need for leadership to focus on system design and also on organisational and inter-organisational development. This becomes particularly relevant in the newer context of 'world-class commissioning'.

Some research (Mintzberg, 1978; McDaniel, 1997; Salaroo and Burnes, 1998) suggests that approaches to leadership and management need to be different where the context is a dynamic rather than stable environment. So leaders may need to adapt their style to different contexts of system change and also to the different kinds of challenges that are encountered. For example, different leadership styles may be more effective at different phases of a merger (further details in Chapter 5 on the challenges of leadership), that is, shifting the leadership approach according to the external or internal context during the change process (Dickinson et al, 2006).

The internal organisational context

Leadership in healthcare also takes place, of course, within discrete organisations (such as hospitals, GP practices, PCTs). From an organisational perspective, this is the internal context. Organisational context here refers to aspects of geographical location, history, size, structure, culture, staffing, skills and resources. The internal environment of the organisation will offer both strengths and weaknesses in relation to the leadership challenges, and as such is an important part of the context for the leader to 'read' and understand.

Brazier's (2005) review of the literature on the influence of organisational contextual factors on healthcare leadership focuses on the power and influence of leaders and their capacity to encourage creativity and innovation. She concludes that bureaucratic organisations can be the most inhibiting for innovation, tending to foster transactional leadership approaches. Hierarchical structures, high staff turnover and tightly controlled resources are most likely to stifle creativity and innovation. On the other hand, she found that organic structures (that is, with high levels of lateral communications, a relatively flat hierarchy, with work teams brought together flexibly to deal with tasks and with decentralisation of decision-making – Burns and Stalker, 1994) facilitate a more transformational leadership approach.

In a study of the contribution of leadership to sustained organisational success in NHS Foundation Trusts, Bailey and Burr (2005) examined the extent to which organisational history and inherited organisational capabilities (which they termed 'legacy') are a significant factor. They define 'legacy' as the long-term impact of eight performance-critical organisational elements:

- the structure of the trust
- the prevailing culture
- technological capability
- operational capability
- quality of staff
- clinical reputation
- strategic relationships
- strategy.

They suggest that effective leadership both builds on and works with the organisational legacy. In other words, leadership rarely starts from scratch but has to work with the existing internal context.

Scott et al (2003) and Mannion et al (2005) highlighted inadequate or inappropriate leadership as a key factor that may impede cultural change within healthcare organisations. These studies stress the importance for leadership of assessing the alignment between organisational culture and the wider environment, including possible 'cultural lag' or 'strategic drift' in achieving alignment. Scott et al (2003) propose an integrated leadership style (both transactional and transformational) to achieve culture change. They suggest that, in developing a patient-centred model of healthcare, the leadership task is about substantially reshaping attitudes and behaviours that can be deeply ingrained in the organisation, through its culture.

Several studies point to the importance of understanding the organisational context, particularly organisational culture, for successfully leading change. Examining the role of senior leaders in implementing quality and safety improvements in healthcare, Øvretveit (2005a) concludes that leaders' actions are important but that their influence as individuals is limited. He proposes a 'system of leadership for improvement', which takes account of where and how leadership can be enabled and demonstrated throughout the organisation, especially by medical leaders. He suggests that senior leaders "need to build a system of leadership for improvement which includes all formal and informal leaders, teams and groups which support improvement as part of the everyday work of an organization" (p 423). In order to do this effectively he argues that "the first step in leading improvement is to understand the organisation's stage of quality development, any internal experience with quality methods and assess 'readiness for change … [as well as] the current pressures which help and hinder improvement" (p 424). In other words, organisational diagnosis is an important aspect of leadership context.

Policy and practice implications:

- A key prerequisite for effective leadership is the need to understand the contexts in which leadership is exercised. Policy-makers, managers and professionals may find it helpful to think in terms of the three layers of context that are outlined here: the national public policy context; the regional and local strategic context, including partnerships; and the internal organisational context.

- These are not discrete levels but interact with each other in complex ways. Systems thinking helps to reveal the interdependence between the elements and to act as a reminder that outcomes may not always be predictable.

- Contingency approaches suggest that different leadership styles are effective in different contexts. Selecting leaders to match particular contexts, and/or helping leaders to develop and deploy particular leadership styles according to the particular context are both important skills to develop.

- 'Reading the context' is therefore a crucial skill. It includes being able to take an overview and link the big picture with the fine-grain detail. Moving between 'the balcony and the battlefield' is one way to achieve this.

- Leadership may involve not only shaping the context but also, in some situations, constituting the context. Leaders have a role in defining and articulating the key points of the context, framing it for others inside and outside the organisation.

- The context for healthcare is changing, due to rising expectations, new illness and disease profiles and the greater emphasis on 'predict and prevent' rather than react and ameliorate. The leadership challenge is to transform and improve, but this requires accurate and careful reading of the context.

- Reading the context of partnerships and inter-professional and inter-organisational networks is a critical skill for healthcare leaders, particularly but not exclusively at senior levels.

- Partnerships may have collaborative advantage but also collaborative disadvantage, so reading the context accurately and thinking through the challenges of partnership working become crucial. Leadership in this context needs to focus on whole-system design and development, to ensure that partnerships contribute to strategic purpose.

- Reading the internal organisational context includes thinking about the strengths and weaknesses of geographical location, history, size, structure, culture, skills, resources and reputation. Leadership has to work with the history of the organisation and its culture and rarely starts from scratch with a blank sheet. Organisational diagnosis is a key element of leadership and the starting point for improvement and reform.

CHAPTER 5

The challenges of leadership

In this chapter:

We examine the challenges, or purposes, of leadership. What is it that leadership is trying to achieve?

First, we examine the challenge of 'sense-making' – how do leaders make sense of the context and the purposes they are trying to achieve, and how do they communicate this to others to create a clear sense of common purpose? We examine 'big picture sense-making' and then turn to consider the different types of problems that leaders may face, and the degree of match between their leadership strategies and the problem, or challenge, to be addressed. How do leaders think about and orchestrate the work to be done? We distinguish between technical and adaptive challenges (sometimes called tame and wicked problems) and the leadership approaches that seem to be most effective in tackling each of these two types of problem.

We then turn to examine five concrete leadership challenges for healthcare organisations. These are: the merger/acquisition challenge; leading partnerships and networks; leading organisational turnaround; leading organisational change, innovation and improvement; and nurturing future leaders in the organisation.

This chapter focuses on the challenges and purposes of leadership (see Figure 5.1). What are the goals or outcomes that leadership is aiming to achieve? We have called these tasks 'challenges' in line with an emerging literature that frames leadership purposes in this way (Heifetz, 1994; Heifetz and Laurie, 1997; Burgoyne et al, 2005; Morrell and Hartley, 2006). Most definitions of leadership focus on purpose in some way – for example, leadership as being influence towards a common goal, or mobilising others to tackle tough problems. The definitions of leadership from Stogdill (1974) or Smircich and Morgan (1982) are a reminder that the leader's role may also be to find or frame the purpose not just to implement agreed goals, or communicate a vision to others.

Figure 5.1: The challenges of leadership

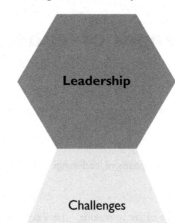

Leadership as sense-making and as constituting challenges

Leadership theory from the 1980s onwards has revived interest in leadership as providing 'vision' and a sense of clear purpose and direction for an organisation or group of followers (for example, Conger and Kanungo, 1987; Nadler and Tushman, 1990; Bryman, 1992). Yet vision is not a simple read-off from the context. Some have argued for a more constitutive approach that is based not only on rational analysis but also on an analysis of the various stakeholders and their interests and an attempt to negotiate a coalition and common purpose. A constitutive approach is about the active framing of what the problem is as well as what the solution is (or rather, perhaps, the range of ways of addressing the problem) (Parry and Bryman, 2006; Heifetz et al, 2009). DuPree (1998, p 130) argues that "The first responsibility of a leader is to define reality. The last is to say thank you". How are purposes formulated, articulated and debated? The complex context of healthcare makes this a particularly fertile site for the exploration of purposes and the contestation of purposes by different stakeholders. In particular, for public services such as healthcare, there is also the question of assessing whether or not the leadership purposes contribute to, or detract from, the creation of 'public value' (Moore, 1995; Benington and Moore, 2010), that is, the wider public good. (Public value is discussed in detail in Chapter 7.)

Grint (2005b) notes that a key element of leadership is to define and make sense of context. The strategic leadership of change is not just a matter of rational decision-making (however persuasive the post hoc rationalisations of leaders may be). Complex change in an uncertain world can only be partially predicted and planned for by the leadership (Hartley, 2000). 'Sense-making' becomes important in organisational change, particularly under conditions of uncertainty or ambiguity (Weick, 1995). Sense-making captures the idea that people (individuals or groups) make sense of confusing or ambiguous events by constructing plausible (rather than necessarily accurate) interpretations of events through action and through reinterpretation of past events. The role of the leader, in a sense-making framework, may be less about being fully clear about the future and rational plans for shaping it (that is, providing a 'clear vision'), and more about providing a plausible narrative that helps people understand what may be happening and mobilises their support and activity to address the problem. Pfeffer (1981, p 4) argues that a key role for leaders is to provide "explanations, rationalizations and legitimations for activities undertaken in organizations". In this sense, the view of leadership as sense-making for and with the organisation is particularly valuable (Smircich and Morgan, 1982; Hartley, 2002b), and this has been noted in relation to healthcare (Weick et al, 2002).

Some writers have formulated purposes, or challenges, at a fairly high level of abstraction, which is helpful for broad orientation but requires more detailed working out in practice. Storey (2004) sets out three key 'behavioural requirements' or meta-capabilities for leadership, which can be seen as part of the key challenges for leadership. An adapted version of his approach is shown in Figure 5.2.

Big picture sense-making aims to scan and interpret the environment, particularly the external political and policy context (analysing context is discussed in Chapter 4 and here we examine how this has an impact on the purposes pursued by the leadership). Another important element of leadership is the ability to communicate the vision, mission and strategy to others, and to help them to make sense of the experiences they have (Hackett and Spurgeon, 1996). In Figure 5.2, inter-organisational representation requires the ability to lead with influence rather than formal authority. The ability to foster organisational and cultural change is the third element of the triangle. This is particularly important in healthcare organisations, given the pace, scope and scale of change both as a response to demographic and social changes and as a response to governmental policy pressures and directives.

Figure 5.2: Three key challenges for leadership

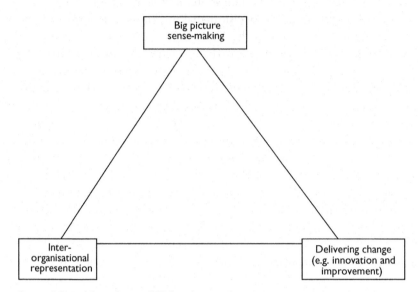

Source: Adapted from Storey (2004)

A different but relevant framework for considering the challenges of leadership comes from Leach and Wilson (2000, 2002). While their work is based on the challenges for local political leaders, it also has resonance for those tasked with strategic management and corporate leadership. Leach and Wilson have formulated four key tasks for elected political leaders:

- maintain political cohesion
- develop strategic policy
- exercise external influence
- ensure task accomplishment.

They note that it is hard, if not impossible, to achieve all of these purposes to the same degree and there are inevitably trade-offs between these challenges.

This framework requires some 'translation' into a managerial or clinical leadership setting, but the first task is recognisable in both settings as building up, consolidating and maintaining a sufficiently strong coalition of support for the proposed policy, direction or purpose. It reminds us why 'ownership' of change is such a widely used concept when organisational and cultural change is embarked on, because if there is insufficient support then the leadership will not achieve its goals (Iles and Sutherland, 2001; Burnes, 2004). Increasingly, support needs to be mobilised outside as well as inside the organisation (Hartley et al, 2007).

Senior leaders will have to spend time in developing strategy, or will be involved in shaping local policy to fit with national policy. Reyatt (2008, p 154) notes that strategic visioning, as a key element of developing policy, involves at its core "imagining what is not present and what should be". Other elements of strategy involve creating concrete plans and actions from that imagination and vision. Westley and Mintzberg (1989) argue that central to strategic leadership is the ability to take account of context but also to work with vision. Kaplan (2006) warns against lopsidedness: the need to link strategy with operations and not just be concerned with strategic ideas.

Exercising external (inter-organisational) influence through partnerships and networks is increasingly important for all types of organisations across all sectors and a key challenge for health professionals, managers and board members. This challenge is covered in more detail later in this chapter.

Task accomplishment is the fourth challenge in Leach and Wilson's framework, and involves making sure the job gets done well once the vision or direction has been established. Strategic leaders have to ensure that this happens, mainly by working through others, rather than through micromanagement.

An ever-present challenge for leadership in healthcare is to create and chart the course for the achievement of organisational goals and objectives. From national performance targets (for example, treatment waiting times), to local priorities (for example, GP prescribing policy), effective leadership has to take account of the many contextual layers and mobilise support for both the approach and its implementation. This in itself will often require leaders to question the status quo, take thought-through risks and search for opportunities (Kouzes and Posner, 1995).

The nature of the challenges

A number of writers have distinguished different types of problem or challenge and argued that they call for different types of leadership. For example, Stewart (2001) distinguishes between 'tame' and 'wicked' problems (Rittel and Webber, 1973) in local government, and Grint (2005b) also draws on this distinction in his analysis of different types of leadership appropriate for different problems. 'Tame' problems include those that have been encountered before, for which known solutions already exist, and which can be addressed by a particular organisation, profession or service. Tame problems may be complicated but they are potentially resolvable through existing practices. The leadership challenge is to make it happen. One example of a tame problem in the health service is the need to wash hands to prevent the spread of infection within hospitals. Everyone knows and agrees what needs to be done – the challenge is to make it happen in practice. By contrast, 'wicked' problems have no agreed diagnosis (different people may formulate the problem in different ways), the solutions are not fully known or agreed, yet there is pressure to resolve the problem in some way. Solving a wicked problem may throw up other challenges because the problems are cross-cutting and interrelated. Often, large groups of people have to contribute to solving the problem, through changing their behaviours. An example of a wicked problem is tackling the health issues of childhood obesity.

A similar distinction is made by Heifetz (1994, 2004), who distinguishes between 'technical' and 'adaptive' problems (equivalent to tame and wicked problems) faced by leaders. We examine these two approaches to challenges because they have major implications for leadership strategies, styles, processes and behaviours.

Grint's typology introduces a third type of problem – a critical problem where immediate and urgent action is needed (for example, dealing with major road traffic injuries in the accident and emergency [A&E] department) and where the people involved in the crisis accept a command and control style of leadership in order to take urgent action, in a way which they would not if there were not a crisis.

Heifetz (1994) argues that technical problems, where the problem or task has been encountered before and the parameters are known, can be dealt with through technical leadership (Grint calls this management). It is the leadership required to bring together resources, people and schedules to deal with the challenge, sometimes in a project-based way. By contrast, adaptive problems (Grint calls these wicked problems) require a different kind of leadership in which the leader must refuse to collude with the fantasy that he or she has magic solutions to the problem and instead must persuade 'followers' that they may need to be involved in addressing the problem and may indeed be part of the problem as well as part of the solution. The leadership challenge in these circumstances is to confront the complexity of the problem and seek to orchestrate the work of a range of people to address it. The idea that different types of challenge may require different types of leadership is captured in Table 5.1.

Table 5.1: Types of problem and forms of authority

Type of problem	Form of authority
Tame problems (technical challenges): Complicated but resolvable Likely to have occurred before Limited degree of uncertainty	*Manager:* Manager's role to provide the appropriate processes and resources to solve the problem
Wicked problems (adaptive challenges): Complex and often intractable Novel with no apparent solution Often generate more problems No right or wrong answer, just better or worse alternatives Huge degree of uncertainty	*Leader:* Leader's role to ask the right questions rather than provide the right answers, because answers may not be self-evident and are likely to require collaborative processes
Critical problems: A crisis situation Urgent response needed with little time for decision-making and action No uncertainty about what needs to be done	*Commander:* Commander's role to decisively provide the answer to the problem

Source: Adapted from Grint (2005b)

While this framework is useful for leaders seeking to understand the nature of the problems or challenges they face, and how to employ different forms of authority to deal with them, Grint's (2005b) analysis suggests that leaders in decision-making mode may be inclined to legitimise their actions "on the basis of a persuasive account of the situation" (p 1475) rather than concluding that effective decision-making necessarily lies in the correct analysis of the situation. Providing a narrative to others that helps to define the situation (as a crisis or not, as tame or not and so on) is one element of leadership, and reinforces a challenge for leadership in both being able to read the context and also to constitute the context. This is not leadership responding to contingency, but leadership framing the reality as seen by others.

The constitutive and perceptual nature of the problem is also captured in the idea that a problem may be seen differently by different stakeholders. What is a crisis to a patient arriving at A&E may be a technical problem to the emergency team who have dealt with this kind of situation many times before. Part of the skill of leadership is in understanding how others frame the situation and then taking that framing into account.

The work of Heifetz (1994) is particularly relevant for thinking about the leadership of complex and cross-cutting problems, where neither the means nor the outcomes are clear or agreed upon. His work is valuable not only in terms of framing and addressing the challenge, but also in terms of challenging the ways of working with various stakeholders involved in the problem – identifying the adaptive challenge; creating a safe but challenging holding environment; regulating the distress; maintaining disciplined attention; protecting the voices of leadership from below; moving continuously between the balcony and the battlefield – see later for detailed discussion of these. Benington and Turbitt (2007) have tested ways in which leaders can address complex or uncertain challenges using adaptive leadership in a very complex policing situation in Northern Ireland – the Drumcree demonstrations:

> Heifetz's theory of adaptive leadership (Heifetz 1994) argues that a distinction needs to be made between technical problems (where there is a general agreement about the diagnosis of the problem, and about the nature of the action required to solve it) and adaptive problems (where there is uncertainty, confusion or disagreement about the nature of the problem, and about the action required to tackle it). He argues that adaptive problems require a different kind of leadership from the tackling of technical problems – leadership which rejects the pressure from followers to provide magical solutions to complex problems, and instead works with stakeholders to take responsibility for grappling with these problems and for the changes in one's own thinking and behaviour that are required. (pp 383–4)

Heifetz outlines a framework of seven principles for adaptive leadership:

- Identify the adaptive challenge – the leader needs to think hard about what the real underlying challenges are (which may not be the same as the presenting problem) and also whether the issues can be dealt with by technical or adaptive leadership. Adaptive leadership is indicated where changes in thinking and behaviour (including one's own) are required to grapple with difficult issues.
- Give the work back to the people faced by the problem – avoid the temptation to solve people's problems for them; engage them in the adaptive work and in their taking responsibility for their contribution to the problem and to the change process.
- Regulate the distress necessary for adaptive work. Heifetz notes that where levels of personal or social distress are very high, a society may reach for extreme or repressive measures to try to restore a sense of

order and control, although for an adaptive challenge this may not solve the problem. So authoritative action is likely to reduce distress while inaction will increase it. A wise leader will keep the level of distress in a range in which people can function effectively, paying attention to the issues but not getting overwhelmed – creating and maintaining sufficient heat to keep things cooking, but not so much heat that everything boils over and spoils. This may involve 'cooking the conflict constructively'.

- Create a 'holding environment' in which the painful adaptive work can be done effectively; this can be a physical and/or a psychological space, providing both safety and also stretch and challenge. Heifetz (1994) defines the holding environment as "any relationship in which one party has the power to hold the attention of another party and facilitate adaptive work" (p 105). An adaptive leader needs to think carefully about the physical and psychological space in which adaptive work gets done.
- Maintain disciplined attention to the issues – recognise the seductions of work avoidance and other displacement activity (for example, dependency, projection, fight/flight), and relentlessly bring the focus back on to the primary task, which is the adaptive challenge.
- Protect the voices from below or outside – ensure that all perspectives and interests are considered, that minority viewpoints are taken into account, and that dominant views are questioned and challenged.
- Move continuously between the balcony and the dancefloor (or battlefield in Benington and Turbitt's [2007] term) – in order to combine a helicopter overview of the whole situation and strategy with an understanding of the changing operational situation at the front-line. The balcony view enables the leader to see all the players on the battlefield and also to look out to the horizon to see longer-term issues. The front-line battlefield perspective gives a strong sense of what issues are like on the ground, and what they feel like for the players, which enables the leader to have greater empathy and understanding in order to regulate the distress and lead the adaptive challenge. It also enables the necessary linking of strategy and operations.

Not all problems require adaptive leadership and Heifetz recommends a different form of leadership (technical leadership) for problems that have familiar parameters (similar to Grint's typology of tame problems). Heifetz's work on leadership for adaptive problems is valuable because it is theory-based (working within a Tavistock-type 'open-systems framework') and because he sees the tasks of leadership as including harnessing the commitment and work of the group(s) that are needed to solve the problem.

Moore (1995) describes the importance of public leaders and managers thinking carefully about and aligning three elements that are needed for a successful strategy to create public value outcomes. The three elements of his strategic triangle are public value goals and outcomes (what is the value proposition in terms of adding value to the public sphere; and what does the public most value?); commitment from the 'authorising environment' (have the stakeholders who are necessary to provide or withhold legitimacy and/or support of the public value proposition been mobilised?); and operational resources (are the necessary resources of money, people, skills, technology and equipment aligned behind the public value outcomes?). This is shown in Figure 5.3.

Figure 5.3: The strategic triangle for public managers

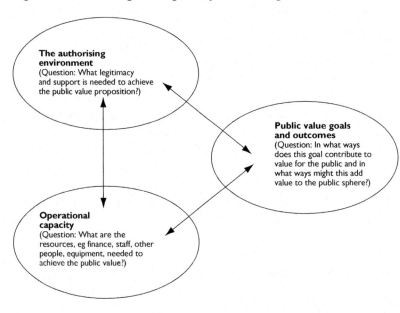

Source: Adapted from Moore (1995)

There are therefore a number of difficult challenges to be juggled by senior healthcare leaders. At a formal, senior level, the leadership role of the chief executive as a non-medical manager responsible for managing an organisation with multilayered and multi-professional responsibilities is complex. According to Blackler and Kennedy (2004):

> [Chief executives] are responsible to government both for the finances and for the clinical performance of their organizations; they must enact national priorities for healthcare and lead local change programmes; develop good working relations with the many professional groups working in their organizations; work with the chair of their board; build relationships with relevant local agencies to develop services for the public and generally foster public confidence in the NHS in line with governmental imperatives. (p 182)

These tasks can be reformulated, in Moore's terms, as being about framing the public value proposition, gaining sufficient legitimacy and support for the approach, and mobilising operational resources (from both within and outside the organisation, through partnerships and networks).

Challenges at the organisational and inter-organisational levels in healthcare

Having looked at how challenges are constituted and framed, we now turn to examine particular tasks/challenges in relation to healthcare improvement, innovation and change. For leaders at every level in the NHS perhaps the biggest challenge is the pace of systemic and organisational change, so here we examine several challenges of organisational and cultural change that are highly relevant in the healthcare field:

- organisational mergers and acquisitions;
- networked or partnership organisational arrangements;
- leading organisations out of failure;
- organisational change, innovation and improvement;
- nurturing future leaders.

The merger/acquisition challenge

The NHS has been through significant mergers (for example, Primary Care Trusts and Strategic Health Authorities) in order to gain claimed efficiencies and to achieve coterminosity with the boundaries of local authorities and the Government Offices of the Regions in England. Research by Dickinson et al (2006) on private sector mergers and their applicability to healthcare has suggested that organisational transition at a time of merger requires particular types of leadership in different phases of the transition period. These are shown in Table 5.2.

Table 5.2: Leadership type related to merger phase

Merger phase	Leadership type
Action pre-merger decision	Transactional: Assess/audit the culture of each of the merging organisations and use this knowledge as part of a careful strategy for highlighting and recognising the differences between the organisations
Decision to merge	Transformational: Create and communicate a vision that sets out the purpose of the transition in an open and participatory manner
During merger process	Transactional: Provide resources to support the change process for staff Manage the human resource and make this your main activity Communicate the changes and latest developments relentlessly Set up clear transitional structures incorporating senior people that enact the transition promptly Attend to sense-making, help staff understand the implications of change
Post-merger	Transactional: Measure the impact of the transition both in relation to transition objectives and other measures – do this for at least three years

Source: Adapted from Dickinson et al (2006)

This research suggests that both transformational leadership (inspiring, transforming) and transactional leadership (practical, operational) need to be used at different stages of the merger transition but that, on balance and perhaps counter-intuitively, a transactional style is the most crucial. (Transformational and transactional leadership types are covered in greater detail in Chapter 6.)

There are, however, particular issues that leaders need to take account of in the merger of NHS organisations that distinguish them from organisations in the private sector. Table 5.3 outlines some of these differences.

In a study of two hospital mergers in Quebec, Denis et al (2001) highlight the challenges posed for leaders in change situations that have been imposed by government and that are often highly contested. They note that:

the challenge of the mergers was not simply one of governance.... Each merger involved the rationalization of activities among the three sites, thus requiring 'micromergers' between myriad clinical services currently operating separately and demanding the fundamental transformation of the mission of some or all of the sites.... Thus, besides maintaining three operating institutions and learning to work collaboratively with former rivals, the leaders had to implement fundamental, [radical] change [which questioned the nature, existence and boundaries of the organization]. (p 828)

Table 5.3: Merger asymmetries between the NHS and the private sector

Private sector	NHS
Acknowledged transition merger process	Merger regarded as closing one organisation and opening another
Potential merger organisations make a choice based on pre-merger assessment and planning	No choice of merger organisation
Possibility of demerging	No possibility of demerging
Organisational differences acknowledged and desirable	Organisational differences not acknowledged
Research shows that mergers do not achieve efficiencies	Belief that merged organisations achieve efficiencies
Focus on merging provider organisations	Focus on merging demand-side organisations
Research shows it takes at least three years for performance to recover after a merger	Mergers tend to follow at about three-year intervals
Empowered providers organise and carve up the system	Commissioning is a weak tool further weakened by reorganisation
Merger processes led by the organisation's board and its directors	NHS merger processes led 'remotely' by politicians
Communication (especially with staff) acknowledged as key to successful merger	NHS poor at communication
Early indications from human resource management that give 'psychological safety' to staff paramount	NHS human resource management processes lead to great uncertainty
The aims of mergers are rarely met	Mergers seen by politicians and policy-makers as a way of achieving policy goals
Mergers are a distraction with negative unanticipated consequences	Front-line staff behaviour is rarely changed as a result of a merger

Source: Adapted from Dickinson et al (2006)

Denis et al conclude that the 'leadership constellation' formed by the integrated board and leadership team for each merger situation needs to reflect the strengths and weaknesses of the historical legacy and 'imprint' of the merging organisations as well as take account of the climate within which the merger is taking place (for example, the degree of political pressure in the external environment and/or opposition to change within the internal organisation). They also suggest that imposed merger situations require transactional leaders able to negotiate and make compromises between different interests and positions rather than the transformational leadership that may be more effective when leading a unified team.

The challenge of leading networked and partnership organisations

Denis et al (2001) explore the strategic challenge for healthcare leaders in 'pluralistic' contexts, where there are diverse interests and priorities within and between partners, and where leadership roles are shared, objectives are divergent and power is diffuse. Their analysis highlights four aspects of strategic leadership in networks and partnerships, emphasising that such leadership needs to be concerned with the network system as a whole. These are shown in Table 5.4.

The researchers concluded that strategic leadership in pluralistic organisations is more likely to be established under unified collective leadership but that this is always fragile in the context of diffuse power. The leadership challenge here is to stabilise the collective leadership as much as possible to prevent it being shattered by internal rivalry (strategic uncoupling), dislocation from the focal organisation (organisational uncoupling) or lack of adaptation to environmental needs (environmental uncoupling). This is an issue that many 'managed clinical networks' are grappling with in the UK.

Alexander et al (2001) also address the issue of collaborative leadership in relation to community health partnerships. They conceptualise collaborative leadership around five mutually reinforcing themes:

- Systems thinking: developing a sound working knowledge of how organisational systems interrelate and affect health at the community level, while also taking into account the big picture.
- Vision-based leadership: communicating a values-based envisioned future, mobilising resources and guiding action towards long-term aims, particularly with key stakeholder groups.

- Collateral leadership: broad-based leadership across the partnership with contributions from partnership staff, organisational representatives and advocates for particular community segments.
- Power sharing: to set priorities, allocate resources and evaluate performance in order to foster a sense of joint ownership and collective responsibility.
- Process-based leadership: translating substantive leadership into action through effective communication mechanisms and good interpersonal skills.

Table 5.4: Aspects of strategic leadership in networks and partnerships

Strategic leadership model	Elements
Collective	Strategic leadership requires contributions from more than a single individual Different individuals contribute in different ways to strategic leadership Recognition of diffuse power, for example, professionals and external agencies Embodied in 'leadership role constellation' or 'top management team' Complementary roles to allow all to contribute in a concerted manner
Action/process oriented	Focus on the actions of people in leadership positions rather than on personality traits Significance of influencing/mobilising others through tactical action
Dynamic	Leadership participants, roles and influences evolve over time Importance of construction, deconstruction and reconstruction of leadership roles Recognition of mutual influence of action and context Significance of the effects of leaders' actions on the organisation, allocation of resources and distribution of power
Supra-organisational	Leadership roles and influences on them extend beyond organisational boundaries Consideration of external influences such as government funding, community, public and political pressures

Source: Denis et al (2001)

Alexander et al's research identifies three challenges that may confront leaders in partnership situations where participation is voluntary. These are set out in Table 5. 5.

Table 5.5: Challenges for collaborative leadership

Leadership challenge	Constraints, trade-offs and conflicts
Continuity versus change	Striking the right balance between maintaining experienced leadership and infusing new leadership into the partnership
Leadership development	Identification of potential leaders, including those within the community but the need to expend considerable effort to orientate them towards the purposes of the partnership and to invite, coach and encourage them to be leaders
Power and participation	Power sharing through 'neutral' leadership that fosters equal voice and representation among all partners and/or 'equity-based' leadership that reflects the financial contribution of partnership members

Source: Adapted from Alexander et al (2001)

The challenge of turnaround and leading organisations out of failure

The UK government's emphasis on performance improvement in public services in the UK, combined with easier and wider access to performance metrics, has made organisational failure both more important and more visible.

Leading organisations out of failure and creating turnaround is a distinctive leadership challenge. Jas and Skelcher (2005) analysed performance turnaround across local government. Like the health service, local government is subject to very public scrutiny of its performance. They found that performance was cyclical (some of the organisations that were deemed by central government to have failed had had very high or very innovative performance in the past). Where awareness of performance decline was absent and where there was low leadership capability, the organisation failed to initiate its own recovery strategy and action, and this led to more authoritarian intervention from central government and its agencies. They also found that building or re-establishing leadership capability required both political and managerial senior leaders to overcome the inertia of failure and to regenerate collective belief across the organisation in its ability to solve its own problems. This suggests that leadership at all levels in the organisation is critical to creating the rapid and major leap forward from what is seen to be failure.

Other authors have examined the choices of turnaround strategies by leaders of healthcare and other organisations, comparing them with the strategies available to the private sector (Boyne, 2004, 2008; Walshe et al, 2004). Boyne (2008) found that turnaround from what had been deemed as failing organisations in health, local government, schools, fire, police and prison services was influenced by the pre-existing context (for example, local deprivation), but also by the ability of the organisational leadership to convince inspectors that appropriate activities had been undertaken and the 'right' systems introduced to create rapid improvement (in other words legitimation in addition to improvement). The leadership challenge is both to face inwards to the organisation to build leadership capacity, and also outwards to manage the reputation of the organisation with key stakeholders.

The challenge of leading change, innovation and improvement

The leadership challenge of developing and sustaining innovation and improvement in healthcare delivery occurs at all levels of the system. Reform, service redesign, re-engineering, improving patient safety and quality, and innovation initiatives may focus on particular techniques and ways of building commitment to sustain cultural change. Nurse managers, doctors and other health professionals, and administrators, as well as senior managers, can all find themselves leading reform and redesign initiatives or aspects of these in projects or programmes of organisational and cultural change.

Research tracking the changing role and responsibilities of nurse leaders in 1993 and 1995, through the American Organization of Nurse Executives network (Gelinas and Manthey, 1997), suggested that organisational redesign had a substantial impact as the US healthcare system shifted from a service for the sick to a service to achieve health, and with a more client-centred, market-responsive structure that required flexible clinical teams. This brought with it different and greater expectations of nurse leaders. The researchers reflect that service redesign often had the following characteristics, suggesting a shift of priorities towards continuity and quality of healthcare, rather than simple cost-cutting exercises:

- integration/coordination across departmental lines;
- critical path/care-protocol development;

- management restructuring;
- multiskilled worker development;
- patient-focused care implementation;
- case management implementation.

Such changes resulted in nurse leaders focusing much more on team-building skills across departmental boundaries, deploying multiskilled workers, as clinical practice was consciously improved. The researchers found that nurse leaders have a critical role in redesign initiatives, with most respondents in the research reporting involvement in both initiation and implementation (although it can be noted that this was as self-reported). Many nurse leaders also found themselves in different reporting relationships and with different formal titles, reflecting a broader role with responsibility for patient care. In most redesign situations, nurse leaders found themselves being required to lead new operational configurations, while reducing costs and also maintaining or improving the quality of care. The challenge here was summarised as the need for nurse leaders to understand how to:

- lead across cultural, functional and departmental boundaries;
- promote teamwork and build and maintain effective teams;
- manage personal growth by objectively challenging their own behaviours and beliefs;
- promote the continued development of the nursing profession in an integrated patient care environment;
- tolerate ambiguity and change.

This research suggests a complex role for nurse leaders:

> Leading clinical improvement across the continuum of care, facilitating integration of clinical services, working effectively with other clinical leaders and ensuring organizational success, are just some of the challenges for current nurse leaders. (Gelinas and Manthey, 1997, p 42)

However, other research carried out in New Zealand found that nurses were not reaching their potential as transformational leaders of organisational redesign due to cultural and social factors in the organisation, linked to traditional, rather limited, conceptions of the nursing role that effectively limited or repressed leadership in the new context (Kan and Parry, 2004). Leadership interacts with the internal organisational context, including its culture, creating both opportunities and constraints.

Systems re-engineering is one major means by which efficiency and improvement in healthcare delivery are striven for. Senior leaders clearly have a critical role to play and need to be equipped to face the challenge. Indeed, lack of effective leadership, including the accurate diagnosis of existing organisational conditions and cultural support for change, has been cited as a primary cause for failure of re-engineering in healthcare (McNulty and Ferlie, 2004).

Guo (2004) suggests that the role of the leader in healthcare re-engineering has four elements that are mutually reinforcing in a cyclical process, as shown in Table 5.6.

Table 5.6: The role of leadership in healthcare re-engineering

Element	Key questions
Examination – of the healthcare organisation and its environment	Timing for the re-engineering process Market challenges and opportunities Organisational strengths and weaknesses Purpose of the organisation Future direction of the organisation Outcomes of the organisation
Establishment – of a long-term strategic plan to determine the direction of the organisation as it deals with the complexities in the environment	Quality Customer satisfaction Cost-effectiveness Improved work environment for employees Realistic goals, timeline and budget Organisational culture and values
Execution – of the strategic plan	Allocation of resources (financial, human, capital) Redefinition of roles and responsibilities Managing conflict Education, training of managers and staff Communication and coordination of work efforts
Evaluation – of desired and unintended outcomes	Reach desired outcomes Effective change for the organisation Continuous feedback to make adjustments Periodic review for more responsive organisation Cooperation, integrated and empowered organisation

Source: Adapted from Guo (2004)

Turning now to consider innovation, a number of writers have argued that, for both the public and the private sectors, innovation is distinct from continuous improvement as a strategy to achieve performance improvement. Innovation may or may not result in performance improvement. Innovation is most usefully seen as a step-change rather than as continuous improvement (Albury, 2005; Hartley, 2005; Osborne and Brown, 2005). The leadership of innovation is likely to be different from the leadership of continuous improvement because the scale and scope of change are different and therefore projects and people may need to be led and managed quite differently.

The particular challenge of the leadership of innovation is the need to be creative and to encourage creativity in others in order to solve problems and generate the energy and enthusiasm needed to overcome inertia (Isaksen and Tidd, 2006). Leadership involves acting as facilitators and educators for change, working to create an environment of 'psychological safety' that fosters risk taking and opportunism, and supports others to learn and adapt their behaviour. Adaptive leadership (Heifetz, 1994) may be one approach to enable others to take ownership of and successfully manage innovation.

The diffusion of innovation is particularly relevant to public service organisations, because many of the benefits of innovation are accrued in terms of policy change at the institutional or sectoral level, in addition to the individual organisational level (Hartley, 2008, 2010c). If a local innovation improves healthcare, there is value in spreading that practice across healthcare organisations rather than the originating organisation protecting its intellectual property. So leadership to support the spread of good or promising practices, through the diffusion of innovation and broader change, is highly relevant to healthcare organisations (Kimberly and de Pouvourville, 1993; Buchanan et al, 2007; Hartley and Rashman, 2007). Such leadership is necessary at both corporate level and at service or team level.

There are many elements in the leadership of organisational and cultural change. Given that change is an ongoing dynamic in organisations, it is an ongoing challenge, or purpose, for leadership at a number of levels in the organisation. Some writers have noted that a key challenge for top organisational leaders is to shape organisational design, organisational culture and the distribution of resources (Senge, 1994; Schein, 2004; Goodwin, 2006). Such leaders, therefore, design the social architecture: "They are responsible for the governing ideas underpinning the policies, strategies and structures which guide business decisions and actions and help build a shared vision" (Munshi et al, 2005, p 12). While this statement was written about the private sector, it is equally relevant for healthcare organisations.

As well as influencing structure, leaders may also have a significant impact on organisational culture. This has been widely reported from the seminal work of Schein (2004) onwards. However, writers vary in how far they see organisations as having a single integrated culture; how far they see a set of subcultures coexisting or competing within the organisation; and how far the sheer size and complexity of large, contemporary organisations means that it is hard to talk about managing or shaping culture in any meaningful way (Parry and Bryman, 2006).

There are many definitions of organisational culture. A useful one is from Schein (1992, p 12):

> A pattern of shared basic assumptions that the group learned as it solved its problems of external adaptation and internal integration, that has worked well enough to be considered valid and, therefore, to be taught to new members as the correct way to perceive, think, and feel in relation to those problems.

The concept of organisational culture is valuable because it reminds the leader that 'message sent' may not be the same as 'message received'. Hatch cautions the leader:

> Do not think of trying to manage culture. Other people's meanings and interpretations are highly unmanageable. Think instead of trying to culturally manage your organization, i.e., manage your organization with cultural awareness of the multiplicity of meanings that will be made of you and your efforts. (Hatch, 1997, p 234)

In supporting change and innovation, there is a task for leadership to create a climate, or culture, which encourages learning from failure as well as from success. Often the ultimate challenge is for leaders to be able to acknowledge defeat in achieving change and innovation! In healthcare systems, one major criticism has been the lack of learning from previous initiatives and the need for leadership to be more reflective. Edmondson (2004) suggests that hospitals do not learn from failure for two reasons. First, because the interpersonal climate at the front-line with patients (reinforced by the professional traditions of medicine) may inhibit questioning and challenge; and, second, because the work design features of hospitals tend towards quick-fix solutions to problems rather than root cause analysis and systematic problem-solving. Other research points to the value of learning from mistakes and unsuccessful attempts at change, as well as learning from successes (Bate and Robert, 2002; Rashman and Hartley, 2002).

The challenge of nurturing future leaders

Some writers also remind us that a further challenge is not only the immediate purpose of goal accomplishment but also building up leadership capacity and capability by nurturing the next generation of leaders and creating a learning approach to leadership (for example, Fullan, 2001; Burke, 2006a). It is about embedding leadership as an integral part of the organisation (Huff and Moeslein, 2004) and fostering the next generation of leaders, both individually through informal coaching and support and formally through leadership development initiatives. Some have called this building a 'leadership engine' (Tichy and Cohen, 1997). This occurs where leaders are seen to occur at all levels of the organisation and where a key role of leadership is actively to develop future generations of leaders, according to Tichy and Cohen (1997). This is about conceptualising the organisation as a system that produces leaders as part of its activities, thereby ensuring long-term capacity and adaptability for the organisation. Many organisations pay insufficient attention to this, either formally through human resource systems or informally through fostering a climate of learning and development for potential leaders.

Policy and practice implications:

- Challenges are partly made not given. A constitutive approach to thinking about the purposes of leadership in any particular context is about the active framing of what the problem is and how it might be addressed.
- Complex change in an uncertain world can only be partly predicted and planned for. Big picture sense-making is an important element of deciding how to address a challenge, or set of challenges. Also important are the challenges of delivering change, and representing the organisation to other stakeholders.
- A key distinction has been made between 'tame' and 'wicked' problems, also described as technical or adaptive problems. The leadership of each type of problem requires different strategies. In the first case, leadership is about bringing together the appropriate skills and resources to tackle a known or solvable problem. The second case involves a complex problem, where neither

---

the causes nor the solutions to the problem are known or agreed. The task of the leader in this case is to orchestrate other people both to recognise their part in the problem and to address ways of tackling the problem together. This can be pressurising for the leader, where the group may want the leader to solve the problem for them, but Heifetz's seven principles (see pp 58-9 above) may help to keep the attention on the problem and promote necessary adaptations in thinking and behaviour.

- Mark Moore's strategic triangle is one means by which healthcare leaders can frame their approach to adaptive problems, by thinking about what is the public value to be created, who can be mobilised to legitimate or support that course of action and how to align operational resources of finance, staff and equipment behind these goals.

- Many of the challenges for healthcare leaders, at whatever level, are to do with bringing about change, whether through mergers, through service redesign, turnaround, or innovation and improvement. Thinking through what the purposes and outcomes are that the leadership is pursuing is helpful.

- Styles or types of leadership will need to vary with the purposes being pursued at any phase of the organisational change. For example, transactional and transformational leadership styles are both relevant at different phases of merger/acquisition.

- Complex organisational change may also be made more effective by relying on a 'leadership constellation' not just an individual leader.

- The leadership challenges of working in networks and partnerships are complex because leadership is generally fragile in conditions of diffuse power. The leadership challenge is to prevent internal rivalry, dislocation from the focal organisation and lack of adaptation to environmental needs.

- Managing turnaround requires the building of leadership capacity and the use of legitimising actions (to maintain the support of external stakeholders) as well as internal activity to overcome inertia and generate confidence to improve.

- Organisational change and improvement is the task of all kinds of formal and informal leaders in the workplace. Some may be constrained by role expectations and organisational culture, suggesting that such changes need to be whole-system approaches.

- Innovation and improvement are different in scope and scale and may require different types of leadership. Innovation requires leaders to empower others to be creative and they have a key role in creating an organisational climate with psychological safety.

- A further challenge for leaders (and one easily squeezed out by other pressures but nevertheless very important) is nurturing future leadership talent so that leaders actively develop future generations of leaders.

CHAPTER 6

The capabilities of leadership

In this chapter:

What are the capabilities (attributes or qualities) of leaders that are most closely associated with effective leadership? The chapter starts by looking at the individual leader and considering the evidence about qualities in terms of traits, behaviours, practices and competency frameworks. The chapter includes a consideration of emotional intelligence and of political awareness as key capabilities for leadership, along with the idea of 'meta-competencies'. The chapter then turns to looking at the behaviours and capabilities of teams (for example across a team, a board an inter-organisational partnership). The chapter then focuses on capabilities in terms of processes of influence between the leader and those being influenced, and, therefore, looks at transformational and transactional leadership, and post-transformational leadership. There is also a brief consideration of the question of gender and the social construction of leadership. This analysis has implications for diversity more generally.

Figure 6.1: The capabilities of leadership

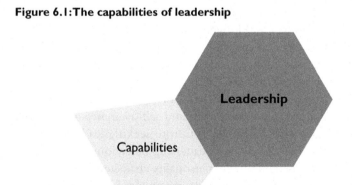

Some leadership writers would put capabilities right at the start of the analysis in this book – so why have we not done this? The individual qualities of leadership might seem a logical place to start ('Who are the leaders and what qualities do they possess?'). It would fit with the tendency that still exists across much of the literature to focus on 'heroic' leadership – the assumption that leaders are different from 'followers' in terms of their special intellect, motivation and/or personality.

However, this book is based on an alternative analytical framework, which argues that the context and the challenges shape the kinds of leaders who will emerge in particular situations, or who will put themselves forward, intentionally or not, as sources of influence. So, this approach is a contingent one, which suggests that the kinds of skills and abilities that an effective leader needs to exhibit will depend on the situation they are in, and the kinds of goals they are trying to formulate or accomplish. We turn now to the evidence about capabilities, within this framework.

Traits

Early research into leadership (up to and into the 1940s) had focused on traits, such as personality, physique and cognitive style. These were assumed to be fixed and largely inherited (Stogdill, 1974). Large lists were generated of the traits that were associated with effective leadership (largely, at that stage, the leadership of small groups).

There were a number of problems with the trait approach to leadership. First, it assumed that leaders were largely born rather than made, because the traits were seen to be innate. Second, however, the list of traits grew longer and longer. Third, this approach did not take into account the different contexts within which leaders carried out their work, which was found to have an impact on leader effectiveness. Fourth, contemporary understanding of personality is that many elements of it may not be fixed but can be developed over time, according to context, life experiences and self-awareness to develop. On the whole, research has moved on from seeking leadership traits to looking at leadership styles and leadership behaviours.

Despite this, a limited number of personality characteristics have been found, in review studies, to be linked to specific leadership approaches. For example, Bass (1998) found in empirical studies of transformational leadership that intelligence, ascendancy, optimism, humour, need for change, behavioural coping, nurturance, internal locus of control, self-acceptance, extroversion, hardiness and physical fitness were related to effectiveness. More succinctly, other research found that "positive, adaptive, developmental and people-oriented traits form a distinct personality pattern that supports transformational leadership's social influence process" (Sosik, 2006, p 41). However, this is based on traits associated specifically with transformational leadership and so may not be relevant to all leadership situations. Overall, the view is that trait theory had very limited applicability to understanding the leadership qualities of effective leaders (Parry and Bryman, 2006; Yukl, 2006; Jackson and Parry, 2008).

Behaviours

Disappointment with trait theory led to a greater interest in the behaviours exhibited by leaders from the mid-20th century onwards. This meant that there was a focus on what leaders do rather than on who they are (in the sense of personality or background). This is also called the style approach, in that it examines clusters of behaviours commonly used by leaders. Here, the focus is still on the individual leader, but examines what can be explicitly seen or sensed through behaviour. It also assumes that behaviours can be acquired, so there is a shift from a dominant interest in selection, to a focus on leadership development.

Early work, such as the famous Ohio studies (for example, Halpin and Winer, 1957), found two key dimensions of effective leadership of small groups. These dimensions were labelled 'consideration' and 'initiating structure'. These reflected behaviours by the leader concerned with consideration for the social and emotional well-being of their subordinates or a focus on shaping and progressing the task. These twin themes of a focus on people and/or task have been echoed in other studies (Marturano and Gosling, 2008) and provide a valuable and recurring framework for thinking about leadership behaviours and styles. These themes have also shaped thinking about leadership development, where a focus on improving personal and interpersonal skills to work with others, and on strategic vision and managerial competencies to address the task, has been important.

Competencies

An important approach to understanding the behaviours of leadership has come from the competency frameworks originally pioneered by Boyatzis (1982, 2006) and widely used both to understand and to improve leadership qualities, though not without critics (for example, Hollenbeck et al, 2009).

A competency has been defined by Boyatzis (1982) as an underlying characteristic of the person that leads to or causes effective or superior performance in a job. More concretely, this has been described as the skills, knowledge, experience, attributes and behaviours that an individual needs to perform a job (or role) effectively (Hirsh and Strebler, 1995). The crucial difference between a trait approach and a competency approach is that the competency approach focuses on qualities that are expressed in terms of behaviour. There is also an assumption that competencies may be acquired (for example, through learning, practice, experience) rather than inherited, as traits are sometimes assumed to be.

Some writers have become rather wary of using the language of competency (as they see it as too rigid and focused on standards and qualifications) and instead use the language of capability. Other writers use the terms interchangeably. Each expresses skills of effective performance whether these are technical skills, interpersonal skills, cognitive skills or broader mindsets and values. (The word 'skill' is often used as a shorthand to cover the range of knowledge, experience, attributes, behaviours and mindsets that make up the qualities that competency covers, rather than the narrower sense of skill as learned behaviours to achieve predetermined outcomes.) Fletcher (2008) notes that a more restricted view of competency is as an observable skill or ability to complete a managerial task successfully. Our focus here is on individual-level competencies not on organisational competencies.

Competencies, or capabilities, are conceptualised as related to job (or role) performance. A competency approach recognises (or should recognise) the interaction between the context and the person. Boyatzis (2006) shows this in a diagram, reproduced as Figure 6.2.

The figure shows the interaction between person and their context, expressed in terms of the job demands and the organisational environment. This recognises that leadership performance is not simply a matter of a particular type of person. This is a contingency view of leadership, in that it is affected by the situation that the leader is in, and is not solely dependent on the qualities of the leader. Boyatzis describes best fit as the "area of maximum stimulation, challenge and performance" (2006, p 122).

Competency frameworks have become a widely used approach in thinking about the qualities for effective leadership. For example, the NHS Leadership Qualities Framework has been widely used in healthcare in the UK and is shown in Figure 6.3. It sets out the key skills or competencies for leaders in healthcare, across a range of settings.

Figure 6.2: Boyatzis's theory of job action and performance

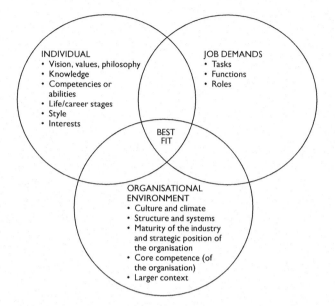

Source: Adapted from Boyatzis (2006, p 122)

Figure 6.3: The NHS Leadership Qualities Framework

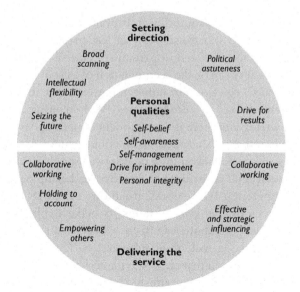

Source: NHS Institute for Innovation and Improvement (2005),
www.nhsleadershipqualities.nhs.uk

Another health example of a competency framework comes from the US, where researchers developed one for those working in public health leadership (Wright et al, 2000). However, this was developed through focus groups and discussion rather than through the more rigorous methodology adopted by Boyatzis, and is based on the idea of a baseline set of competencies rather than the behaviours associated with superior performance as in the Boyatzis model. The public health approach identified four main areas of job demand (challenge) and clarified the competencies required for each of: transformation; legislation and politics; trans-organisation (inter-organisational partnerships and networks); and team and group dynamics.

Some have argued that a competency approach to leadership is restrictive because it creates abstract qualities about leadership (Bolden and Gosling, 2006) and that this applies to the NHS Leadership Qualities Framework specifically (Bolden et al, 2006). On the other hand, Boyatzis emphasised the need to consider leadership competencies in their context, and so it seems that the practice in some organisations is problematic where competencies have been treated as if they can be conceptualised and used on their own, as essential and primary ingredients of leadership (Bolden and Gosling, 2006). In this restricted use, the focus can become blinkered to concentrate solely on the person's individual behaviours, at the expense of understanding the context or the job demands, and their interaction with the organisational purposes and environment. There is a danger that competencies are then used mechanistically for job promotion, job evaluation or development. This can obliterate a situational view of leadership, where effective leadership is seen to be related to particular contexts.

A further difficulty can be the accumulation of a list of competencies, which (like traits?) can grow in number. For example, the US public health framework has 79 competencies (Wright et al, 2000). This becomes unwieldy, and there is a consequent danger of developing an idealised skill set that only a superhuman could achieve. Also, there is a danger of competencies becoming a descriptive list rather than a theory about how such skills contribute to effective leadership performance.

Some competency frameworks are more evidence-based than others – a focus on behaviours helps to make explicit what the practices are that contribute to effective performance and help to anchor performance in real, observed practices. This is in preference to judgements about skill that are not evidence-based but are prone to personal judgements, which are affected by personal biases, attribution errors and halo effects.

Most competency frameworks cover a range of personal, social and cognitive, or conceptual skills. For example, personal skills may include self-awareness, confidence, integrity, resilience in the face of adversity. Social skills might include the ability to empathise with others, to communicate clearly and persuasively, maintaining cooperative relationships. Conceptual skills might include analytical ability, creativity, having foresight, making sense of complexity.

Some elements of leadership capability have received particular attention recently. It is not within the scope of this book to cover them all, but here we look at three specific clusters of capabilities: emotional intelligence, political awareness and meta-competencies.

Emotional intelligence

Emotional intelligence (Mayer and Salovey, 1993; Goleman, 1995) is a concept that suggests that people vary in how far they are attuned to emotional, not just rational, aspects of life. In terms of leadership, emotional intelligence involves awareness of the feelings, moods and emotions of oneself and others, and the ability to act in ways that contribute to goal formulation and goal achievement, taking into account the emotions of those whom one is attempting to influence (Goleman, 1995; Goleman et al, 2002; Dulewicz and Higgs, 2004; Cherniss, 2006). The interest in emotional intelligence provides a counterweight to those theories that had primarily emphasised rational aspects of leadership (for example, analytical ability) and where emotion in the workplace was seen as dysfunctional. Scholarly opinion is divided as to whether emotional intelligence is a distinct capability or whether it is an amalgam of other capabilities (Matthews et al, 2002). It has certainly been useful in alerting leaders to think about and act in emotional terms, not just in rational terms, and to harness emotions constructively in the workplace (Dulewicz et al, 2005). This may be particularly important in healthcare, where staff are working with a range of emotions from patients, carers and others, with their own emotions, and with the consequences of emotion on their own work (Menzies Lyth, 1988; Hoggett, 2006). There is an accumulating body of evidence (for example, Cherniss, 2006), which suggests that emotional intelligence, in a variety of conceptualisations and measured by a variety of tools, does have either a direct impact on leadership effectiveness, or else an indirect effect (for example, a link between emotional intelligence and transformational leadership style, or the organisational commitment of 'followers').

Goodwin (2006) has also suggested that leaders in the NHS would benefit from using emotional intelligence to manage the stress caused by organisational and wider health system change, including managing their own anxiety and pressure. He draws on the Goleman model of emotionally intelligent leadership, which requires personal skills:

- To know what you are feeling and be able to handle those feelings without them wholly dominating your interpersonal relationships and decision-making.
- To be able to motivate yourself to achieve personal and group objectives, to be innovative and creative and to perform at your peak.
- To sense what your team and others in wider networks are feeling and thereby handle interpersonal and inter-organisational relationships effectively.

Leadership with political awareness

Political awareness, political astuteness, political acuity and political intelligence are all terms that cover the ability to analyse and act as a leader taking into account diverse groups that may sometimes compete and sometimes collaborate. The NHS Qualities Framework defined political astuteness as "showing commitment and ability to understand diverse interest groups and power bases within organizations and the wider community, and the dynamic between them, so as to lead health services more effectively" (NHS, nd, p 21).

Recent work by Hartley et al (2007) and Hartley and Fletcher (2008) has examined the key skills of political awareness among senior leaders in the private, public and voluntary sectors in a large, national survey, based on 1,500 managers across the private, public and voluntary sectors, and including a substantial number of managers from healthcare. The political awareness skills framework is based on the recognition that increasingly leaders have to influence a diverse range of individuals, groups and organisations, not only inside the organisation but outside as well, through networks and partnerships, and because of the increasing connectivity and transparency of organisations through information and communication technologies. Leadership with political awareness was found by Hartley et al (2007) to operate on five dimensions: personal skills; interpersonal skills; reading people and situations; building alignment and alliances; and strategic direction and scanning. They found that senior and middle managers reported using political awareness skills in a wide range of contexts, reflecting both 'small p' and 'big p' politics, with managers having to be Janus-faced, that is, facing into and outside the organisation, in order to lead diverse, and sometimes competing, interests among a variety of stakeholders. They also found that managers reported acquiring their political awareness skills through a variety of somewhat haphazard routes, with 88% reporting making mistakes as a valuable or very valuable way of gaining these skills. The research makes recommendations about making development more systematic and less painful, through actions by individuals, organisations and development providers.

One context where political awareness is particularly needed (as found in the research) is in working in networks and partnerships, where both collaboration and competition may coexist (Hartley and Fletcher, 2008). Some UK writers have examined the capabilities for health leaders working in networks. Goodwin (1998) notes that a senior manager such as a chief executive will need to work with, and attempt to influence, a wide range of stakeholders. Ferlie and Pettigrew (1996) found that having strong interpersonal communication skills (including listening skills), having an ability to persuade others, and having an ability to construct and maintain long-term relationships were critical to an effective approach to leading health networks.

Overarching competencies

Finally, in this section, Fletcher (2004) undertook an analysis of the leadership competency frameworks in use by Welsh public service organisations, that is, in use in the NHS Wales, in Welsh local government and in the Welsh Assembly government, as part of a larger analysis of leadership development for the whole public service system in Wales (Benington, 2004). Fletcher found that it was possible to summarise the main strands of competency in terms of eight principal themes, but that there were, in addition, two 'meta-competencies', as identified by Briscoe and Hall (1999). Meta-competencies are overarching competencies in that they enable the acquisition of other competencies. As leaders operate in a dynamic and uncertain world, the competencies that gave effective leadership performance in the past may no longer contribute or contribute as fully to future performance. Therefore, the ability to acquire new competencies becomes crucial. The eight competencies and two meta-competencies that enable the acquisition of further competencies are shown in Table 6.1.

Table 6.1: Analysis of competencies and meta-competencies in Welsh public leadership

The eight core capabilities include skills in:
Motivating, empowering and developing staff, by establishing and communicating high expectations and high standards.
Inspiring, promoting and facilitating change, encouraging new ways of working, influencing perceptions of change – making it achievable and exhilarating.
Providing purpose and vision, translating the vision into practical goals, and ensuring that the longer-term perspective informs and inspires thinking and action.
Establishing credibility and integrity, transparency and consistency, honesty and courage, respect and responsibility.
Influencing and persuading based upon evidence and argument, analysing opposing viewpoints, negotiating, finding common ground, building networks.
Building teamwork and partnerships, encouraging cross-boundary working, seeking diverse viewpoints, empowering stakeholders in decision-making.
Focusing on customers and delivery, identifying customer needs and tailoring the service to meet them, continuously improving performance and outcomes.
Commitment to learning and self-awareness, awareness of one's own strengths and limitations, applying learning from own and other experience.
The two 'meta-competencies' or 'learning competencies', which affect the ability to acquire other competencies, focus on:
Identity – accurate self-assessment; seeking, hearing and acting on feedback; being able to modify self-perceptions as attributes change.
Adaptability – comfort with turbulent change; ability to identify the qualities needed for future performance; and flexibility to make the changes needed.

Source: Clive Fletcher, in Benington (2004)

The capabilities of leading networks and teams

The increasing interest in distributed leadership (Gronn, 2002; Spillane, 2005) means that capabilities shared or distributed across a team or a board, or across the leadership of a group of organisations, is becoming more important. There is still relatively little work on the leadership qualities of whole teams or governance groups, much less research specifically within the health sector.

More broadly, networking has been increasingly recognised as a key skill of leaders. For example, some case study work on collaborative community health partnerships in the US (Alexander et al, 2001) suggests that leadership has a number of requirements in practice:

- the need to think in terms of whole systems;

- to be able to develop, communicate and work with a vision of what is to be achieved, consisting of a core ideology and an envisioned future;
- collateral leadership (which is another way of saying distributed leadership);
- power sharing across a partnership in order to build a broad basis of support;
- process-based leadership, by which the authors mean a set of capabilities that involves the leaders paying attention to how the work gets done as well as what is done.

Denis et al (2005) and Peck and Dickinson (2008) point out that network leadership is not only about interpersonal skills and the ability to build relationships between people, but also about the ability to understand the structural power that pervades such networks, particularly for public service organisations such as health. Denis et al (2005, p 453) note that "In organizations where power is diffuse, success or failure of the strategic process depends, among other things, on the capacity of leaders to constitute and maintain strong and durable networks". This includes the ability to "pull together a powerful alliance with diverse internal and external actors" (p 454) and with the capability to:

> think simultaneously in terms of both the project and the networks of support they can engage. He or she will be drawn to consider the diverse meanings that various project definitions will have for others and how those meanings might be reconstructed either discursively or practically to render them more or less attractive. (p 454)

This ties in with leadership as the management of meaning, and sense-making, as well as the achievement of goals (Smircich and Morgan, 1982; Weick, 1995; Pye, 2005).

It has been noted (Denis et al, 2001, forthcoming) that major organisational change in complex healthcare systems is more likely to happen where there is a 'leadership constellation' in which different individual leaders play different roles or contribute different aspects of leadership at different phases of change, and where leadership roles are constructed and reconstructed as the change progresses. A leadership constellation may be particularly important in organisations with multiple professions, priorities and views (such as hospitals or universities) where a coalition to define, build support for and engage in leadership is critical.

There has been a small amount of work on the capabilities of whole boards, and therefore the competencies required both by individuals and by the whole board for healthcare governance (McDonagh, 2006; Endacott et al, 2008). Some work has suggested that chief executives and chairs have a leadership role to play in ensuring that a focus on clinical care is linked to all trust developments, so that the 'business of care' is considered alongside financial performance (Burdett Trust for Nursing, 2006). This is perhaps an area where further research and development would be helpful.

So far, the focus in this chapter has been on the personal qualities of leaders, whether acting as individuals or in a network or group. The emphasis is on the leader and their behaviours and practices and less about the impact on those whom they are trying to influence. The chapter turns now to examine leadership style in terms of the relationship between leaders and those they try to influence. It is not possible to cover all theories in this field so we have selected for detailed analysis one that has particular prominence in healthcare leadership research, and that is influential but sometimes misunderstood. This is the area of transformational and transactional leadership. We then turn to consider 'post-transformational' leadership as a reaction to this work.

Transformational and transactional leadership behaviours and styles

Theories based on the idea of transformational leadership have become very popular in leadership research and practice in recent years. Transformational leadership is interesting on several counts. First, this approach takes into account not only the skills of leaders but also the impact of leader behaviour on so-called 'followers' (although these are often not the subordinates implied in the word follower, but individuals, groups and organisations whom the leader aims to influence). Second, the theory tries to take into account the situations in which leadership is exercised. Third, it has attracted considerable empirical research, which provides evidence to support many (though not all) of its conclusions. It is an approach that has attracted interest in the healthcare sector, where a number of studies have been conducted. Transformational leadership is part of a cluster of theories linked with charismatic leadership (for example, Conger and Kanungo, 1987; Bryman, 1992), and visionary leadership (Westley and Mintzberg, 1989) based on creating strong links between leaders and 'followers'.

—

Transformational leadership theory has been developed, alongside its apparently contrasting cousin, transactional leadership, from initial research by Burns into political leadership (1978). Transactional leadership is based on an exchange process between the leader and 'followers'. The transaction is based on what the leader possesses or controls and what the 'follower' wants in return for providing their services. The exchange may be economic, political or psychological, and the relationship between leader and follower may involve negotiation as a core component.

Transformational leadership, on the other hand, is based on the leader inducing positive feelings in their followers, which then motivate loyal and committed performance. The leader aims to engage followers in going beyond their self-interest because the leader seeks to win their trust, admiration and loyalty and so they are emotionally as well as rationally inclined to do more than they originally expected to do. The theory of leadership behaviours and competencies has been particularly developed by Bass and colleagues in the US (Bass, 1985; Bass and Avolio, 1990; Avolio, 1999) and Alimo-Metcalfe in the UK (Alimo-Metcalfe and Alban-Metcalfe, 2004, 2005). The latter developed much of the empirical measurement and research with managers in UK health and local government. Nadler and Tushman (1980) have described transformational leadership as 'envisioning, energising and enabling'. In his later work, Bass (1999) outlines four key elements of transformational leadership, which are summarised by Yukl (2006) and shown in Table 6.2.

Table 6.2: Transformational leadership behaviours

Transformational behaviours:
Idealised influence – behaviour that arouses strong follower emotions and identification with the leader.
Intellectual stimulation – behaviour that increases follower awareness of problems, and influences followers to view problems from a new perspective.
Individualised consideration – providing support, encouragement and coaching to followers.
Inspirational motivation – communicating an appealing vision, using symbols to focus subordinate effort and modelling appropriate behaviours.

Source: Adapted from Yukl (2006, p 263), based on the work of Bass (1999)

Transformational leadership has been very fashionable, and it is sometimes assumed that transformational leadership is 'better' than transactional leadership because it rises above a kind of pragmatic, cost–benefit analysis and exchange (transactional leadership) to engage followers emotionally in higher aspirations and goals (transformational leadership). However, while Burns has perhaps implied that transformational leadership is superior, Bass is very clear that effective leaders in practice use both types of behaviour styles. The evidence from research studies shows that the approach varies by context and challenge.

Transactional leadership can sound rather basic, with its focus on exchange, but some have argued that this underestimates the skills of transactional leadership. Being clear, focusing on expectations, giving feedback are all important leadership skills. These are shown in Table 6.3.

Table 6.3: Transactional leadership behaviours

Transactional leadership behaviours:
Clarifying what is expected of followers' performance.
Explaining how to meet such expectations.
Spelling out the criteria for the evaluation of this performance.
Providing feedback on whether the follower is meeting the objective.
Allocating rewards that are contingent on meeting those objectives.

Source: Summarised from Tavanti (2008), which draws on the work of Bass (1985)

Transactional leadership can be particularly effective in hierarchical organisations where the followers are subordinates and where the group is focused on achieving clear task objectives. Transformational leadership may be valuable in dynamic, unstable environments (Yukl, 2006) where there is an accepted need for change and where the organisational or partnership climate is such that leaders are encouraged and given powers to be more entrepreneurial in their approach to the task and their group. Mannion et al (2005) argue for contingent leadership in healthcare organisations: "leadership that is able to express and embody corporate vision, but equally able to follow through with the transactional details" (p 438). Other research has found both transformational and transactional leadership development to be important for the health service (Edmonstone and Western, 2002; Peck et al, 2006). This also corroborates the earlier analysis of transformational and transactional styles in relation to the challenges of leading change (for example, different phases of merger/acquisition, see Chapter 5).

Transformational and transactional leadership have been measured in a variety of ways, particularly through the Multi-Factor Leadership Questionnaire (MLQ) designed by Avolio et al (1990). In the health field, numerous studies have been undertaken with nurse managers, but fewer studies have been undertaken with doctors, or with health service managers (Morrison et al, 1997; Corrigan et al, 2000, 2002; Stordeur et al, 2001; Vandenberghe et al, 2002; Leach, 2005; Aarons, 2006). Transformational and transactional leadership have also been explored using a range of research methods, including case studies, interviews and even experimental studies (based on laboratory tasks), as reviewed by Yukl (2006).

Avolio et al (2004) studied 520 staff nurses in a large hospital in Singapore and found that transformational leaders foster higher levels of identification and commitment to the organisation from employees. This study suggests that where senior leaders create a greater sense of empowerment among staff this can have a positive effect throughout the organisation. This is echoed in a national study of 396 nurses across the US, where higher levels of transformational leadership tended to occur in more participative organisations (Dunham-Taylor, 2000). In addition, drawing on Bass's model, studies carried out on 54 mental health teams at the University of Chicago (Corrigan et al, 2002; Garman et al, 2003) found that transformational leadership seems to be associated with a generalised positive effect on staff, positive views by staff about the organisation and low burnout among staff.

Transformational leadership has been the 'spirit of the age' from the 1990s onwards, and there has been considerable work on its qualities and its impact on subordinates and colleagues. It is valuable as an approach to thinking about the qualities that are advantageous for leadership in health, whether from doctors, managers, nurses or others. It emphasises the need to inspire others with a strategic purpose and to engage with hearts as well as minds. It is a relational view of leadership, that is, it is based on how leaders interact with others, rather than on abstract qualities of the leader in isolation. The approach, by focusing on style, implies that many of the behaviours can be learned, fostered and developed. The focus on empowering others through intellectual stimulation, individualised consideration and so on means that it can help organisations to think about the 'leadership pipeline' as well as existing leaders, that is, helping to foster the next generation of leaders.

However, there have been some criticisms, and some of these are particularly relevant to public service organisations such as those in healthcare. First, researchers have noted that different versions of transformational leadership appear to emphasise different clusters of behaviour and this is particularly true of transactional leadership (Yukl, 2006). Second, Kelloway et al (2005) note that transformational and transactional leadership are not discrete categories and that any leader may display some behaviours from each approach. Both of these issues might be problematic for healthcare leadership development if the leadership model is either not understood or not clearly specified. Third, there has been little exploration of how the characteristics of leadership, which were explored in Chapter 3 (roles, sources of authority, and power and resources), interact with leadership behaviours. It could be that different sources of authority may lead to different uses of transformational leadership – one could imagine this being the case for the leadership behaviours of medical consultants compared with chief executives, board members or nurses, or doctors compared with patient representatives. Fourth, transformational leadership theory is so fashionable that it may be held up in some quarters as 'the answer' to all problems and situations, although the research evidence is more contingent, favouring both transformational and transactional leadership according to context and purpose (as noted earlier in this chapter and in Chapter 5).

Fifth, one element of transformational leadership is 'idealised influence', that is, behaviour that arouses strong follower emotions and identification with the leader. This element derives from the interest in charisma as an element of leadership, which is based on the belief among followers that the leader has unusual and valuable gifts. Arousing strong emotions can be problematic on several counts, particularly in public service settings. Public services are provided under a political mandate from government so there are inevitably tensions around how far leadership can or should be based on charisma rather than policies. In addition, the attribution of exceptional powers and abilities to the leader can undermine a group's sense of its own empowerment and abilities, setting up unhealthy dependencies on the leader. This is one aspect of the 'dark side' of leadership theory (Buchanan, 2003; Burke, 2006b) and this has fostered interest in post-transformational leadership. Furthermore, there can be problems with charismatic leaders especially in closed environments, such as psychiatric wards and children's homes, where power asymmetries can become abuses of power. For these reasons, while the theory of transformational leadership is promising, it also has some limitations.

Post-transformational leadership

There has recently been a shift away from the focus on transformational leadership (Parry and Bryman, 2006). The series of corporate scandals such as at Enron showed the limits of transformational approaches. Storey (2004, p 32) notes that "a common trait in the charismatic leaders studied was their willingness to deliberately fracture their organizations as a means to effect change". There has been recognition of some of the darker elements of transformational leadership in some situations, including narcissism and arrogance.

The theory of adaptive leadership by Heifetz (1994) is a valuable antidote to the view of the exceptional leader as charismatic, because he argues that leaders often have to be able to disappoint the expectations of their 'followers' that the leader will solve all problems for the group. Heifetz argues that adaptive leadership is based on enabling the group to accept and address the issues it is responsible for, thereby rejecting inappropriate dependency on the leader. Fullan (2001) argues for an approach to leadership that is based on supporting learning in others across the whole organisation rather than taking on heroic problem-solving.

What about gender?

Debate continues to bubble about whether women are different from men in their leadership capabilities (eg Alimo-Metcalfe, 1999). Behind the debate are questions of evaluative judgement (better or worse). A recent review of the literature concluded that "there is no consensus in the literature about gender differences in leadership styles" (Parry and Bryman, 2006, p 461). Women are only slightly more likely than men to use transformational leadership (see, for example, Eagly et al, 2003), despite the common assumption that women are more relationship-oriented than men.

However, people do hold stereotyped beliefs about 'natural' gender styles and these could influence how people behave at work. For example, it is often expected that women will be more nurturing, and this could encourage women to place more attention on interpersonal relations at work. There is also evidence that the stereotype of the 'heroic' leader is closer to a typical male set of traits than a typical female set of traits, and this explanation has been used to explain why there are fewer women managers (Schein et al, 1996) and fewer women leaders (Sinclair, 2005) in the workplace. Thus, the views about the talents of women or men may be less to do with their inherent qualities and quite a lot to do with the way that society views leadership.

These findings are also relevant in relation to diversity more generally. For example, there is a significant under-representation of black and minority ethnic (BME) managers in senior positions in the NHS. Understanding how leadership is socially constructed and may disadvantage particular groups in society is an important area but one that appears to be under-studied.

Policy and practice implications:

- Capabilities refers to a range of skills, knowledge, experience, mindsets, attributes and behaviours that are associated with superior performance.
- It is helpful to think not about universal qualities of leadership, but what works, in what kind of role and in what kind of situation.
- The search for personality traits has turned out to be limited beyond a few features. It is more useful to think about leadership in terms of behaviours and styles (clusters of behaviours).
- The shift from traits to behaviour also implies that leadership capabilities can be developed. Leadership development comes to the fore as a way to create future leaders.
- Competency frameworks are most useful where they consider behaviours related to the job demands (the challenges of leadership) and what is needed in a particular organisational environment. Leadership performance is not simply a matter of a particular set of competencies.
- Emotional intelligence has captured the interest of policy-makers and practitioners because it emphasises the need to understand one's own and others' emotional states and capacities. It counterbalances more rational approaches to leadership that have focused on analytical skills. Both may be important.
- Leadership with political awareness is emerging as an important set of skills, as leaders at a variety of levels have to understand and work with diverse stakeholders inside and outside the organisation, both locally and nationally.
- There is increasing interest in the competencies that enable leaders to acquire new competencies. These meta-competencies or learning competencies include accurate self-assessment and being comfortable with change and challenge.
- Thinking not only about the capabilities of individuals but also of teams, groups and boards becomes increasingly important in the context of more distributed leadership and more complex challenges.
- Although transformational leadership is popular, the research evidence shows that both transformational and transactional leadership make important contributions to leadership, and that each may be relevant to different situations or different phases of leadership.
- There is increasing caution about the charismatic element of transformational leadership (arousing strong follower emotions) in public service (and other) settings. There is interest in 'post-transformational' leadership, which is focused on creating a climate of organisational learning.
- There is sometimes speculation that women make better (or worse) leaders than men. The research evidence on gender differences is very weak. So it is

not helpful to assume that women (or men) have particular leadership styles. This is valuable for thinking about diversity more generally.

- There is evidence of gender stereotypes in relation to leadership, which may help to explain the fact that there are fewer women managers and leaders in top jobs.

CHAPTER 7

Consequences of leadership

In this chapter:

The ideas and the evidence about how leadership has (or is thought to have) impacts on other people and on organisational and health outcomes is examined. It is widely asserted that leadership is critical for organisational performance whether in the public, private or voluntary sectors. But what is the evidence? We examine the problems of establishing the impact: lack of data; lack of clear causation; and attribution errors. The chapter then looks at two frameworks that may help to tease out the impacts, or consequences, of leadership. Yukl's framework focuses on three organisational impacts: efficiency and process reliability; human resources and relations; and innovation and adaptation. The chapter then takes a broader view of consequences by using a public value perspective to look at outcomes and impact. Evidence from healthcare is then examined in relation to this framework, focusing on inputs, activities, partnership/network working and co-production, user satisfaction, outputs and outcomes.

Figure 7.1: The consequences of leadership

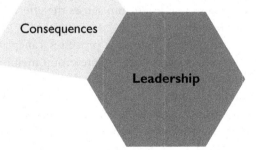

Establishing causes and effects

There are any number of texts that assert that leadership is critical for organisational performance, whether in the private, public or voluntary public sectors. In the public sector in the UK, there has been a particular emphasis on leadership as one of the means by which improvements in services and/or service transformation is achieved. Leadership was signalled as central to the reform of UK public services, with the Cabinet Office's Performance and Innovation Unit document *Strengthening leadership in the public sector* (PIU, 2000). There was no escape from the prevalence of leadership in public service reform under the Labour Government from 1997 onwards. Health is no exception to this, and the Darzi report (DH, 2008) pays particular attention to the need to develop leaders, both clinical and non-clinical, in order to improve healthcare.

However, while the impact of leadership on performance is often asserted, the evidence is more fragile, ambiguous or incomplete. There are problems on several fronts in relation to evidence. First, there is more writing about leadership in general descriptive terms than there is detailed research evidence. Some of this is 'the romance of leadership' (Meindl and Ehrlich, 1987). So, it is sometimes claimed that particular qualities, behaviours or practices are relevant for 'effective' leadership but no data are given. This leaves the field open to broad principles and vague generalisations that are not supported by evidence. Second, some writing is vague about how 'effectiveness' is defined – what is the outcome that influential leadership is expected to produce? What concrete indicators and/or measures of performance are associated with effective leadership?

Third, leadership is often assumed to result in improved outcomes, implying that there is a causal link from leadership to outcomes. However, many studies are cross-sectional in nature and while leadership may be associated with the outcomes, such research designs are unable to establish that leadership causes the effects or to rule out alternative explanations.

Furthermore, attribution errors or processes can play a part. For example, it is possible to have cases where group members assume or believe that leadership is effective because there are positive outcomes, or they assume the existence of leadership because of positive outcomes. These are illustrations of reverse thinking in terms of causation – a type of attributional misinterpretation (Cha and Edmondson, 2006; Martinko et al, 2007).

The idea of charismatic leadership hints at attributional error, because 'followers' may project extraordinary or exceptional qualities onto the leader when they have positive experiences. There are also situations where the attribution is the opposite – where 'followers' attribute negative qualities to the leader when a situation does not meet expectations (Bion, 1961; Cha and Edmondson, 2006). Thus, attribution can lead to disenchantment with the leader despite the leader's best intentions. Psychodynamic theories also emphasise leadership-performance attribution in terms of the internal psychological processes of the 'followers' and the unconscious processes of the group (for example, Bion, 1961; Hirschhorn, 1997; Kets de Vries, 2006).

Finally, there may also be situations where the leadership is so subtle or so participative that commentators are not aware of the full extent of the leader's role in achieving outcomes. The saying of the Chinese master, Lao-Tzu, is a reminder of this: "But of a good leader who talks little when his work is done, his aim fulfilled, [the people] will say: We did it ourselves" (Lao-Tzu, translated by Bynner, 1944, sentence 3).

As we explored in Chapter 6, there can be different attributions about leadership effectiveness depending on whether the leader is male or female (Ford, 2005; Sinclair, 2005; Parry and Bryman, 2006). This is not about whether women *are* different as leaders but whether they are *seen to be* different and judged accordingly by those they come into contact with and try to influence.

How people construct meanings from leadership acts, roles, contexts and experiences affects whether and how leadership is seen to be effective. Leadership and leadership effectiveness is socially constructed, not simply read off from actions and behaviours. The quality of the relationship between the leader and the people being influenced, and the organisational, cultural and policy context, may all shape whether leadership is viewed as effective. This also means that the evaluation of leadership and leadership development is not straightforward.

With these caveats in mind, we now turn to consider two frameworks that may help to think systematically about potential impacts of leadership.

A framework linking leadership and organisational performance

Yukl (2006) unpacks the potential impact of leadership on organisational performance, setting out three major strands, or meta-categories, of the potential impact of leadership and these are shown in Table 7.1.

Table 7.1: Management systems, programmes and structural forms for improving performance

Efficiency and process reliability
Performance management and goal setting initiatives (for example, management by objectives, target setting, zero defects)
Process and quality improvement initiatives (for example, lean management, six sigma, the productive ward, quality circles)
Cost reduction initiatives (downsizing, outsourcing, budget restructuring)
Structural design (reorganisations, commissioning arrangements, service reconfiguration)
Appraisal and rewards linked to efficiencies and process reliability
Human resources and relations
Quality of work–life initiatives (flexitime, job-sharing, child care, fitness centre)
Employee benefits (terms and conditions, sabbaticals, study leave)
Socialisation and team-building (induction, ceremonies, social events and celebrations)
Staff development (continuing professional development, education, training, 360 degree feedback)
Human resource planning (succession planning, recruitment initiatives)
Empowerment initiatives (self-managed teams and collaboratives)
Appraisal and reward linked to service, skill or skill acquisition
Innovation and adaptation
Needs analysis initiatives and environmental scanning (for example, health needs in particular populations and subgroups, policy analysis)
Market analysis (intelligence to inform commissioning, benchmarking; competitor products and processes; international comparisons of healthcare services and processes)
Innovation initiatives (creativity development, entrepreneurship, piloting and testing)
Knowledge acquisition (ideas from a range of sources, promising practice ideas, evidence-based practice)
Organisational learning (knowledge management systems, seminars and workshops; debriefing, learning from near-misses in clinical practice; developing models of learning, use of organisation development managers and leads)
Temporary structural forms for implementing change (for example, steering committee, task force, diagonal slice of staff)
Growth and diversification initiatives (preparing for Foundation Trust status, building clinical specialities, strategic commissioning, joint ventures)
Appraisal and rewards linked to innovation and patient satisfaction

Source: Adapted from Yukl (2006, p 371) to incorporate examples of current initiatives in the NHS

Yukl elaborates on each strand by looking at the activities that can be used by leaders to develop organisational (or team or service) performance. Impacts may occur not only through direct interaction with colleagues but also indirectly through having an impact on organisational systems, which themselves may shape individual, team and organisational performance. The table is valuable for being one of the few accounts that systematically maps the range of possible impacts. It suggests how a leader can judge their own impact or that of others in leadership positions.

A public value perspective

The Yukl framework is valuable when considering consequences of leadership for organisational performance. But a public value perspective (Moore, 1995; Benington and Moore, 2010) may be helpful in thinking about the consequences of leadership beyond organisations, and upon citizens and communities, and society as a whole. Public value is a theory of particular relevance to public service organisations such as healthcare, where the impacts may be much broader than the individual or the specific organisation and that may benefit – or detract from – the wider community and society. For example, reducing the risk of diseases in the community, preventing climate change, building public trust and confidence in the healthcare system are all outcomes that contribute benefits to the public sphere. In addition, some public organisations also have a role to play in establishing collective rules and purposes (Marquand, 2004).

Applying these ideas to healthcare, it is possible to think about the value created not only by activities and services to treat illness and disease, but also the contributions that healthcare can make to illness prevention, and to a societal culture in which people take responsibility for many aspects of their health through their lifestyle choices. A public value perspective becomes increasingly important as the UK health service aims to shift more into 'predict and prevent' rather than just 'treat', and into the promotion of well-being (Tritter, 2010).

Benington (2010) defines public value as having two elements: "what the public values" and "what adds value to the public sphere". The first part of the definition means taking account of the expressed needs and aspirations of users of services, their advocates, and citizens and taxpayers and complementing this with the judgements of the producers. This is an argument to take into account the views of the public, in its myriad forms, but goes beyond what the public 'wants' and focuses more questioningly on what the public most 'values'. This involves the making of trade-offs and choices between competing priorities. The second element of the public value definition is "what adds value to the public sphere":

> This counterbalances the first part of the definition ("what the public values") by focusing attention not just on individual interests but also on the wider public interest, and not just on the needs of current users but also on the longer term public good, including the needs of generations to come. (Benington, 2010)

Public value is one approach to conceptualising the consequences and outcomes of public services. The concept originates from Mark Moore in the US (Moore, 1995) but is now being further developed by Benington and several other academics in the UK, Europe and Australia (for example, Alford and O'Flynn, 2009; Benington and Moore, 2010). Ideas about public value have been applied in the UK to the BBC, to further education, to policing and to the health service (Benington et al, forthcoming).

The consequences of leadership can be conceptualised by using a model of the public value stream, shown in Figure 7.2. This examines all the processes through which value is added via the various stages of inputs, activities and processes, outputs, user satisfaction and outcomes. The attraction of value stream analysis is that it enables the added value of a public service such as healthcare to be assessed at each stage, identifying those processes that add value, those that subtract value and

Figure 7.2: The public value stream

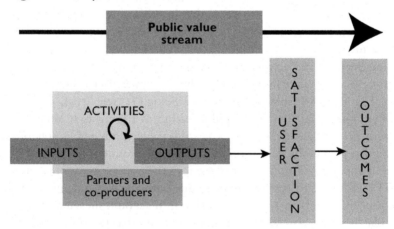

Source: Diagram from Benington and Moore (2010)

those where public value is stagnant. A key question for leadership is whether and how leadership can contribute to the public value stream and generate added value for the public sphere.

Examining healthcare from this perspective, leadership could potentially contribute at a number of points, as follows:

- *Inputs:* How leadership (and leadership reputation) might influence recruitment and selection of staff, financial resources available to the organisation, equipment and technological resources, other inputs.
- *Activities:*
  - How leadership impacts on the activities that take place within the healthcare organisation, for example, systems and procedures, team-working, improvement and innovation initiatives, organisational and cultural change, organisational capacity and adaptability.
  - How leadership has an impact on the attitudes and practices of staff within the organisation.
  - How leadership contributes to organisational capability and capacity (including the 'leadership engine' mentioned in Chapter 5).
  - How leadership can have an impact on the co-production of health working with patients, families, partner organisations and communities. Part of the leadership role may be to help patients to understand where they can contribute to their own health outcomes rather than just relying on health professionals (for example, medicine compliance, following health advice, thinking about preventative health actions through lifestyle).
- *Outputs:* How leadership shapes the outputs of the organisation, for example, the number of operations undertaken, the quality of healthcare advice, the proportion of the population screened or immunised and so on.
- *User satisfaction:* How leadership influences patient and public satisfaction, and the satisfaction of those who are carers for patients (for example, families, relatives, health advocates).
- *Outcomes:* How leadership has an impact on health outcomes more broadly, for example, prevention of future illness, trust and confidence in medical practitioners among the population and so on.

Public value outcomes may be examined from a number of stakeholder perspectives – both internal (for example, doctors, nurses, managers) and in terms of external stakeholders such as the government, the local authority health scrutiny panel, advocacy and patient groups and so on. They may not always agree on some elements of impact. Public value outcomes are inevitably contested and are subject to continuous debate and challenge, through formal political channels, the media and in teams, organisations and communities.

Evidence of the impact of leadership on organisational performance and on health outcomes

It is often asserted that leadership has an impact on the group being influenced and on organisational performance but it is important to turn to the evidence to know:

- whether a causal, correlative or no relationship exists between the leadership and the performance outcome;
- what specific aspects of leadership contribute to the impact;
- how the impact is thought to happen;
- whether the impact is direct (for example, immediate impact) or indirect (through other variables);
- what contingencies or features of the organisational or wider context affect whether leadership is effective or not.

We will explore the empirical evidence using the public value stream framework.

Inputs

There are few studies about the impact of leadership on organisational inputs. Anecdotally, there is a view that inspiring or effective leaders attract good staff to work with them, but more robust evidence is hard to find.

An interim report by Bailey and Burr (2005), based on consultation with chief executives, found that these leaders estimated that about 20% of leadership success in acute trusts was due to 'legacy' – that organisational performance was partly due to the organisation's history rather than the current situation. Part of this legacy might be presumed to be the previous leadership. Recent work about senior management in the university sector (Goodall, 2009) suggests that the choice of leader is affected by the type of previous incumbent – for example, there is evidence of a pendulum swing between the appointment of academic and managerial types of vice-chancellor. Both pieces of research are a reminder that leadership rarely starts with a blank canvas, but must take into account recent organisational history, current organisational culture as well as size and other organisational factors.

Activities

This section examines the impact of leadership on staff attitudes to work, attitudes to work practices, attitudes to improvement and innovation, and the use of scientific evidence in health professional practices.

The idea that leaders have an impact on the attitudes and behaviours of the staff they directly supervise has been established since leadership studies began. In relation to the health service, a number of studies have examined leadership approach and job attitudes among nurses. For example, Morrison and colleagues (1997), in a survey of US nurses, found that both transformational and transactional leadership styles correlated with job satisfaction but that transformational leadership had a greater impact on empowerment (as the theory would predict). Other studies have reported that transformational leadership is associated with higher levels of self-reported job satisfaction, satisfaction with the leader, organisational commitment, work effort and reduced intention to leave the job (Taunton et al, 1997; Vandenberghe et al, 2002; Borrill et al, 2003). Other work in health has found that transformational leadership is associated with lower levels of burnout, specifically emotional exhaustion, among nurses, but also that some aspects of transactional leadership are associated with positive outcomes including assigning tasks, specifying procedures and clarifying expectations (Stordeur et al, 2001). In fact, at the unit level, transactional leadership more than transformational leadership was associated with perceived unit effectiveness (Vandenberghe et al, 2002). These findings reinforce the view, examined in the capabilities chapter (Chapter 6), that both transformational and transactional leadership are important. This also underlines the need for good management as well as good leadership in many organisational settings.

An unpublished paper by Borrill et al (2003) reported a large study that involved over 23,000 staff across 134 UK trusts (acute, specialist, primary care, mental health and ambulance). They found that both top management leadership and direct leadership (immediate supervision) were associated with staff well-being (as measured by overall job satisfaction and low intention to leave the trust). However, the relationship was much stronger with direct leadership, suggesting that it has a particular impact on staff attitudes towards their work. This may be a reminder of the value to staff of daily and direct engagement with, and influence by, leaders.

All of the studies reported are based on cross-sectional data (data collected at the same time) and so it is not possible to say that leadership causes staff attitudes to work. However, work outside health has suggested that there may be a causal relationship, based on research conducted over time (Arnold et al, 2007; Nielson et al, 2008; Barling et al, 2009).

Having examined work attitudes, what is the impact of leadership on work practices? These include behaviours related to improvement and innovation in the workplace, and also the use of evidence-based practices in healthcare.

Two studies (Laschinger et al, 1999; Manojilovich, 2005) found that leadership that encouraged empowerment and self-efficacy (belief in one's ability to be effective) among nurses was also associated with a higher level of professional practice. Research with mental health providers (Aarons, 2006) found a relationship between transformational leadership and the willingness of staff to voluntarily adopt evidence-based practice. However, willingness to adopt was also influenced by aspects of the internal organisational context such as policies and procedures. There were also individual differences related to education and experience.

A large study by West and colleagues (2003) about leadership, team processes and innovation in healthcare found that leadership had an impact on innovation but that the relationships varied by type of team and organisational context. The study examined healthcare teams made up of a range of different professionals (for example, GPs, nurses, administrative and managerial staff, specialist doctors and nurses, medical consultants and so on). Leadership had the potential to influence four key team processes: clarifying objectives; encouraging participation; enhancing commitment to quality; and support for innovation. Leadership clarity was associated with better team processes, and with actual innovation – and ambiguity about leadership was associated with low levels of innovation. This supports the role of leadership in helping to create a compelling direction and ensuring participation of team members in decision-making. However, interestingly, leadership clarity was associated with innovation for community mental health teams and breast cancer teams, but not for primary care teams. Given that the latter are more often varied in team composition, with less clear team boundaries and roles, there may be an effect of group composition, type of task and degree of clarity about leadership, so it is not only about the leadership approach.

A key review of the impact of leadership on quality and safety improvement was undertaken by Øvretveit (2005a, 2005b). He notes that "although most literature emphasises the importance of committed leadership for successful quality and safety improvement, research evidence supporting this is scarce and often scientifically limited" (2005a, p 413). However, from the evidence that is available he concludes that senior leadership is critical for improvement, so long as those senior leaders have a strong commitment to quality improvement and demonstrate this through their behaviour. Examples of demonstrating commitment include taking stock of quality improvement programmes and being flexible about how they are introduced on the basis of encouraging learning from their introduction on the ground. Other studies have reported a lack of leadership as being critical to poor attitudes to quality improvement. Involvement of the board and of doctors by senior managers is also important (Weiner et al, 1997).

Other roles are also important in improvement – including middle managers, doctors and other health professionals, and also 'opinion leaders', that is, those whose opinion is influential with colleagues: "Engaging doctors is essential to quality improvement" (Øvretveit, 2005a, p 422). The variety of roles involved in improvement suggests that creating organisational systems and a climate that supports improvement is valuable.

Øvretveit argues for the need to consider the impact not just of individual leaders but of a system of leadership for improvement that includes "all formal and informal leaders, teams and groups which support improvement as part of the everyday work of the organization", where leaders for improvement are "any people who influence others to spend time on making the service better for patients" (Øvretveit, 2005a, p 423). This requires thinking about organisational capacity and organisational processes.

Finally, Barrett and colleagues (2005) argue, from their study of regional health authorities in Canada, that in complex organisations there is a need to see leadership as one of the important foundations for organisational learning, and for leadership to promote practices that support and enhance organisational learning. They found a clear relationship between leadership and such capacity-building.

Partnerships and co-production

There is relatively little evidence about the role of leadership in partnership working (in terms of working across organisations and in networks). There is some anecdotal evidence and some suggested frameworks for evaluating partnership, or collaborative advantage, in healthcare (for example, Lasker et al, 2001; Dickinson, 2009; Glasby and Dickinson, 2009), but less actual evidence at this stage about the impact on either organisational practices or outcomes.

Co-production is the idea that some (not all) services are created by the interaction of 'producers' (for example, in the case of health, doctors, pharmacists) and 'consumers' or clients (for example, in the case of health, patients, carers) (Alford, 2009). The service cannot be effective in terms of health outcomes unless there is a willing, capable and attentive patient or patient advocate. So the impact of leadership on encouraging the recruitment and engagement of patients, community representatives and others in the co-design and delivery of healthcare could be important. There are examples of trust leadership encouraging, for example, the involvement of newly arrived refugees in supporting the health activities of others in their own language and cultural communities. Public and patient involvement is one element of co-production. Experience-based design is starting to gain ground in healthcare (Bate and Robert, 2007) and shows the impact of leadership on designing and achieving change.

Patient satisfaction

Evidence of the impact of leadership on patient satisfaction and patient outcomes is hard to come by, perhaps in part because the impact of leadership is likely to be indirect (mediated through the actions of staff and the quality of systems of healthcare). In addition, patient satisfaction can be influenced by expectations and other factors, so is not always a reliable or valid indicator of quality services.

A study of managerial leadership in just over 200 US hospitals found that senior management is more strongly linked with process quality than with clinical quality: "hospital management has more influence on process design, improvement and execution than on clinical quality, which is predominantly the doctors' domain" (Marley et al, 2004, p 362). On the other hand, Goodwin (2006) comments that poor leadership has a greater impact on patients than on staff, although he does not provide research evidence to support this conclusion.

Work by Shipton et al (2008), however, provides some hard performance data, including patient complaints as a percentage of treatments, trust star ratings (the former national rating system for trusts) and Commission for Healthcare Improvement (CHI) clinical governance review ratings. The sample included over 17,000 staff and 86 trusts. The research found that staff ratings showed that better senior leadership was associated with fewer patient complaints.

Outputs

Outputs can be examined both directly (for example, tests and operations performed) and indirectly (through external audit and inspection regimes). Some research shows that the impact of leaders on overall organisational performance is through shaping or influencing the culture (and some of the subcultures) of the organisation or the climate for quality care. Mannion and colleagues (2005) used a research design of two high- and four low-performing hospital trusts in the UK (based on star performance ratings in the national rating system) and then carried out case studies of their functioning, including leadership and management orientation. Their analysis suggested that high and low performance environments may be very different environments in which to work, suggesting considerable cultural divergence. Interestingly, they found that the leadership in high performance trusts tended to be characterised by top-down 'command and control' styles, with strong directional leadership from the centre and a 'top-down' approach to performance and organisational change. In contrast, the four trusts deemed to be low performing (with new turnaround management teams brought in because of the trusts' 'underperformance') had leaders who were widely seen to be charismatic. But they were seen to lack the transactional leadership skills needed to create and maintain effective performance management systems.

Additionally, in the low performers, the use of emotional engagement through charisma meant that loyalty to the senior management team was highly valued – but that the organisations seemed to have a monoculture with insufficient questioning and exploration as a result, and with an 'emasculated' middle level of management. There was a focus on internal functioning but insufficient attention to the demands from the external environment, and an over-dominance of clinical interests in decision-making. This is a small but detailed case study project, which raises important issues about the relationship of leadership style to the task in hand, and the influence of the external context on the leadership challenges (see also Scott et al, 2003). Research by Shipton et al (2008) found that senior leadership was associated with a strong emphasis on quality healthcare (which they called 'the healthcare climate') and this was related to the performance of the trust as measured by the star ratings used at the time.

Buchanan (2003) argues that, when designing leadership development, it is important to consider organisational effectiveness from a number of different angles, in order to avoid being trapped in a particular leadership style. He suggests that the balanced scorecard by Kaplan and Norton

(1996) is one way to try to ensure a rounded view of performance and could be applied both to individual organisations and to those that promote and provide leadership development.

Outcomes

Evidence on the relationship between leadership inputs and healthcare outcomes at the societal level is hard to find. The need to think about the wider purposes of healthcare organisations in terms of public value outcomes should help to create a valuable agenda for future research. The leadership of large, complex but effective healthcare organisations is not just about the number of patients treated, but is also about how to contribute to happy, healthy communities and societies.

A contingency view of consequences

This chapter has reviewed the 'consequences' of leadership, while also noting that attributions affect what is perceived as leadership and its consequences. There is less hard evidence than there are claims about the impacts of leadership upon performance at team, service, staff and patient, and organisational levels. Nevertheless there is some evidence that leadership can have an impact on these elements, although there is a need for much more information about how and why leadership has these impacts.

There is also a need to understand more about the contingencies of effective leadership. What are the environmental contexts or organisational conditions that promote or inhibit the relationship between leadership influence and practical outcomes? This chapter has shown that some aspects of leadership are associated with positive outcomes in some settings and some tasks. Certain types of leadership (for example, direct or indirect, technical or adaptive, with or without authority) are more closely associated with certain types of outcomes than others.

The evaluation of leadership impact therefore needs to be based on 'what works for whom, when, how and why' rather than on universalistic principles. It was noted earlier that a key skill of leadership is 'reading' and analysing the context and this may be crucial for thinking about how best to create positive consequences for staff, patients, the organisation and for wider public value.

Policy and practice implications:

- The idea of causal consequences of leadership is provisional in that there is relatively little in the way of longitudinal evidence of its impact.
- In addition, perceptions of leadership effectiveness and leadership impact are shaped by attributions (how people explain what is cause and what is effect). These may not be accurate but can be firmly held. This can underestimate the impact of leadership by women (and probably minority ethnic leadership too).
- Effective leadership may not be noticed or commented on – a consolation for the leader who has worked hard but who does not receive appreciation!
- In terms of organisational performance, strategic and operational leaders may wish to reflect on how far they are able to have an impact on efficiency and process reliability, on human resources and human relations, and on innovation and adaptation.
- A wider public value perspective also considers the impact of the healthcare organisation on the public sphere.
- The public value chain is one useful way to conceptualise the potential impact of leadership on healthcare: through the impact on inputs, activities, partnerships and co-production; on patient and carer satisfaction; on outputs; and on outcomes.
- Different stakeholders may not agree on elements of public value that are created. The impact of leadership is not an exact science.
- There is a fair degree of evidence that leadership can have an impact on staff attitudes. Both transformational and transactional leadership can contribute to job satisfaction but transformational leadership seems to have a greater impact on a sense of empowerment.
- Direct leadership is particularly significant for staff attitudes.
- The impact of leadership is also affected by organisational context, including type of task, type of team, organisational culture and roles.
- Leadership has a substantial role to play in creating organisational climates that support patient safety and a commitment to quality improvement.
- More effective senior management is associated with fewer patient complaints.
- While there has been a strong fashion for transformational leadership, research on leadership style and trust ratings suggests that transactional leadership can be important for creating and maintaining effective performance management systems.
- There are arguments for adopting a multifaceted approach to measuring the impact of leadership. The public value chain is one approach, the balanced scorecard is another.

CHAPTER 8

Leadership development

In this chapter:

The implications of this review for how leaders and leadership are developed are examined. We return to the 'Warwick Six C Leadership Framework' and use each of the elements to inform thinking and practice about leadership development, drawing on the previous chapters on concepts, characteristics, contexts, challenges, capabilities and consequences and using these to critically think about, design and evaluate leadership development practices. The chapter defines leadership development and presents a framework for comparing how far leadership development is focused on individuals and how far it is focused on teams, groups or organisational capacity. The framework also presents a continuum from intentional development (for example, education and training programmes, mentoring) and emergent development (for example, job challenges and hardships). The implications for selecting staff for leadership development opportunities, for designing leadership development, and for evaluating leadership development are explored.

Figure 8.1: Leadership development

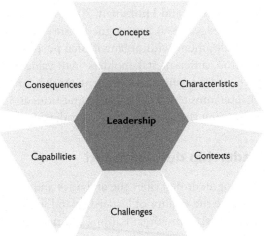

The Six C analytical framework, presented at the beginning of this book, is now used to examine leadership development. Figure 8.1 shows the same structure of elements of leadership but with leadership development rather than leadership in the centre of the figure. In other words, the Warwick framework is used to reflect on how the understanding of leadership affects thinking and practice in relation to leadership development. Leadership development is a large area in itself, deserving greater space than a single chapter (for example, Hartley and Hinksman, 2003; McCauley and van Elsor, 2004; Mabey and Finch-Lees, 2008; Gold et al, 2010). The focus here is limited to particular implications of the framework for selecting staff for leadership development, the design of leadership development and the evaluation of leadership development.

This book has reviewed some key literature about leadership – what, then, are the implications for leadership development? Research (for example, Alimo-Metcalfe and Lawler, 2001) shows that leadership development is often embarked on with insufficient attention to the implicit or explicit model of leadership that is being used, and without attention to the evidence about 'what works' in leadership development. There is sometimes an implicit belief that leadership development is 'a good thing', without clear objectives and without clear planning to ensure that it fits with the strategic direction and priorities of the organisation, or that it is supporting relevant skills and values, that it is efficient and effective in resource terms, and contributes not only to individual development but also to organisational change and improvement.

There is sometimes also a view that there is a 'right' or 'best' (universal) approach to leadership development. A number of writers (for example, Buchanan, 2003; Hartley and Hinksman, 2003; Burgoyne et al, 2005; Benington and Hartley, 2009) have argued instead for the alignment of leadership development with organisational purpose, practices and people. In addition, different stakeholders may value and emphasise different aspects of leadership development (Mabey and Finch-Lees, 2008). This chapter aims to ask appropriate questions about leadership development by using the Warwick Six C Leadership Framework.

What is leadership development?

Leadership development describes the activities and experiences that are used to enhance the quality of leadership and leadership potential in individuals, groups, teams, organisations and networks.

Traditionally, the emphasis in leadership development has been on formal training and education programmes. While these are still important, there has been increasing recognition that a wider range of knowledge-generating activities, including formal and informal, intended and emergent, activities and experiences, can be very formative in developing the skills of leadership (McCauley and van Elsor, 2004; Burgoyne et al, 2005; Benington et al, 2008).

Rodgers et al (2003) provide a typology for both leadership development and its evaluation. Their first (horizontal) dimension is based on the extent to which leadership is focused on developing the individual or on developing collectives (for example, teams, boards, distributed leadership, shared leadership). The second (vertical) dimension is based on the extent to which leadership is prescriptive or emergent. Prescriptive approaches to leadership development can design the inputs (for example, skills, competencies, traits and so on) or the outputs (for example, standards, performance) required for leadership (and therefore leadership development) in particular organisational settings. By contrast, emergent approaches to leadership development view leadership as a dynamic process, with a set of interactions between leaders, followers, context and so on, and therefore that leadership has properties that arise from these interactions and that cannot be predicted in advance. The combination of these two dimensions provides four quadrants of leadership development (and leadership development evaluation), as shown in Figure 8.2.

Figure 8.2: A framework of leadership development

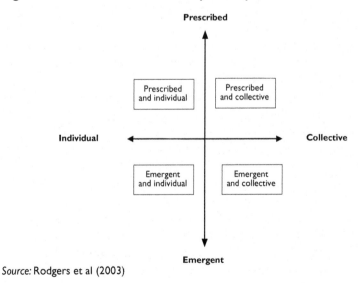

Source: Rodgers et al (2003)

This figure is a reminder that leadership development can be achieved in a range of ways, both formal and informal, focused on the individual or the group. So, leadership development may consist of a range of initiatives including formal training courses, psychometrics, fast-track cohorts, job experiences, coaching, secondments and so on.

The concepts of leadership

Chapter 2 on the concept of leadership noted that leadership is often assumed rather than defined, and that there are a variety of ways of conceptualising leadership. A number of writers have warned of the difficulties for leadership development that can arise if the model of leadership is not clear, or if the approach to leadership is based on following fashion rather than promoting a purpose. For example, Alimo-Metcalfe and Lawler (2001) found that the definition of leadership was nebulous and ill-defined in the 30 organisations they studied and that this is problematic for leadership development for a number of reasons. Without a clear and agreed approach to the conceptualisation of leadership, leadership development practices may be inappropriate for the kind of leadership outcomes that the organisation is aiming for (for example, developing transactional leaders when the organisation needs transformational leaders), or old and outdated practices may be relabelled as 'leadership' to suit the current rhetoric. In particular, if the leadership development designers are not clear about where the boundaries lie between leadership and management then some leadership development may actually confuse the situation and lead to reduced performance because it is really traditional management development (Rost, 1998). Alternatively, in the 'rush to leadership' (Rodgers et al, 2003), courses may be designed to enhance a diffuse understanding of leadership where actually practical management skills may be more fit for purpose.

It was noted in Chapter 2 that clarifying the relationships between leadership and management can be important, given the degree of confusion between the two concepts and the varied ways in which they are used. Day (2001) suggests that:

> Leadership development is defined as expanding the collective capacity of the organizational members to engage effectively in leadership roles and processes.... Leadership roles refer to those that come with and without formal authority, whereas management development focuses on performance in formal managerial roles. Leadership

processes are those that generally enable groups of people to work together in meaningful ways, whereas management processes are considered to be position- and organization-specific. (p 582)

He notes an overlap between leadership development and management development, but suggests that management development tends to focus on enhancing task performance in management roles, whereas leadership development involves building the capacity of individuals and teams to help staff learn new ways of doing things that could not have been predicted.

On the other hand, too rigid a distinction between leadership and management can be problematic: "erecting this kind of dichotomy between something pure called 'leadership' and something dirty called 'management', or between values and purposes on the one hand and methods and skills on the other, would be disastrous" (Glatter, 1997, p 189).

Some balance is needed in clarifying the distinction between leadership and management, while also recognising the degree of overlap (see Figure 2.2 in Chapter 2). It is possible to characterise leadership as the compass and management as the map – both are needed in conjunction with each other on difficult journeys.

Chapter 2 distinguished between the person, the position and the process as approaches to the concept of leadership. There can be value in considering how to develop the skills and resources of persons. However, if the concept of leadership is a 'heroic' one – that is, about exceptional individuals – then there is a danger that leadership development will focus on personal development to the exclusion of, for example, analysis of the context, or leading with others. It runs the risk of focusing more on selecting the 'right' people, that is, people with exceptional gifts or exceptional potential, for development opportunities, rather than widening the opportunities for development across a group or organisation.

If the concept of leadership is about position, then there may be a focus in leadership development on providing opportunities to those in specific ranks or roles. This can be valuable in that leadership is likely to vary according to level in the organisation and scope of the post. However, if leadership development is entirely about those in formal positions, there may be a lost opportunity to think about how to develop informal leaders within and outside the organisation.

If leadership is thought of as a set of processes between individuals, groups and organisations, then leadership development activities may be focused on activities that enhance influence and mobilisation skills. But a focus on 'process' alone may create a rather lop-sided approach to leadership development, which under-emphasises context, roles or resources.

Thus, clarification of the conceptualisation of leadership being used in any given setting is an important prerequisite for effective leadership development. This is an important issue for commissioners and providers alike.

The characteristics of leadership

In Chapter 3, it was noted that leadership characteristics may vary according to the role (for example, degree and type of authority; whether the people to be influenced are near or distant to the leader; the degree to which professional expertise is relevant to leadership). Leadership development activities need to be geared to the roles and resources of those in leadership positions. For example, where a leader is a 'near' leader, with daily interaction with those they influence, then the focus may be particularly on the interpersonal and social skills of influence. Where the leader is 'distant', leadership development may need to focus in addition on how to influence people indirectly through strategy, communicating the vision, and thinking about how to have an impact on the organisational culture and systems. For clinical leaders, different skills need to be developed as they move from clinical practice to clinical leadership (Clark et al, 2008) and this needs to be factored into the design of the programme.

Chapter 3 also considered how far leadership is seen as an aspect of a leadership constellation (Denis et al, 2001), shared or distributed leadership, or leadership configuration (Gronn, 2009). This may affect the approach to leadership development. Day (2001) makes the distinction between leadership development programmes that aim to build human capital (individual leaders), and those that aim to build social capital (leadership as shared within a group or community):

> Leadership has been traditionally conceptualised as an individual-level skill. A good example of this is found in transformational leadership theory which proposes that transformational leaders engage in behaviours related to the dimensions of Charisma, Intellectual Stimulation, and Individualized Consideration.... Within this tradition, development is thought to occur primarily through training individual, primarily intrapersonal, skills and abilities....

These kinds of training approaches, however, ignore almost 50 years of research showing leadership to be a complex interaction between the designated leader and the social and organizational environment.

In addition to building leaders by training a set of skills or abilities, and assuming that leadership will result, a complementary perspective approaches leadership as a social process that engages everyone in the community.... In this way, each person is considered a leader, and leadership is conceptualized as an effect rather than a cause.... Leadership is therefore an emergent property of effective systems design.... Leadership development from this perspective consists of using social (i.e. relational systems) to help build commitments among members of a community of practice. (p 583)

While the conceptual distinction between leader development and leadership development is a useful one, both types of development are important, according to the context and the needs of the organisation. The implications for leadership development are spelt out by Day (2001) and shown in Table 8.1 overleaf.

The increasing recognition of the value of distributed leadership (Bennis, 1999; Bennis et al, 2001; Gronn, 2002) suggests that leadership development may be effected in part through organisation-wide initiatives, not just programmes for individuals (O'Connor and Day, 2007). This suggests that if leadership is partly about organisational change, then situations of organisational change and development may help to foster leadership skills and the social capital of leadership. There may also be the need to think about cohorts learning and developing together (Benington and Hartley, 2009), such as the fast-track and/or graduate entry cohorts that have been developed in health, in central and local government, and in policing (Hartley and Hinksman, 2003). Increasingly, in order to improve services in a joined-up way, there is also a need to think about leadership development as joined up across, not just within, services (Benington and Hartley, 2009), such as in the Leicestershire Leadership in Partnership programme run with Warwick Business School.

Overall, leadership development requires careful thinking about who is to be developed, and what their potential roles and contributions are within and for the organisation. Different types of leaders use different sources and processes of influence, and it is helpful for leadership

Table 8.1: Human capital and social capital approaches to leadership development

Comparison dimension	Development target	
	Leader	Leadership
Capital type	Human capital	Social capital
Leadership model	Individual Personal power Knowledge Trustworthiness	Relational Commitments Mutual respect Trust
Competence base	Intrapersonal	Interpersonal

Skills	Self-awareness
	  Emotional awareness
	  Self-confidence
	  Accurate self-image
	Self-regulation
	  Self-control
	  Trustworthiness
	  Personal responsibility
	  Adaptability
	Self-motivation
	  Initiative
	  Commitment
	  Optimism
		Social awareness
		  Empathy
		  Service orientation
		  Political awareness
		Social skills
		  Building bonds
		  Team orientation
		  Change catalyst
		  Conflict management

Source: Day (2001)

development to be designed appropriately. Some focus may be on individuals, some may be on a whole team, unit or organisation. The exact balance will depend on any given setting, and will also relate to the contexts and the challenges, covered in the next sections of this chapter.

The contexts of leadership

The growing recognition of the importance of analysing context means that leadership development that helps people to 'read', understand and interpret the existing context, patterns of change and potential future scenarios is particularly important (Glatter, 2004; Mole, 2004; Leach et al, 2005).

Chapter 4 argues that the context, in the case of healthcare, is not just the internal NHS organisation but also the wider political and economic context and the strategic context of the health economy. Effective leadership development needs to be able to help leaders and potential leaders to understand and work with a complex, adaptive whole system. The context also includes the growing need to work with other organisational partners and inter–organisational networks, so there is a need in the NHS for leadership development across sectors, services and levels of government, where sharing and comparing across organisations is seen as a key element of the leadership development approach.

Developing the skills of 'leadership with political awareness' is relevant to enhancing skills in 'reading' and interpreting context. Political awareness skills have, until recently, been developed primarily on an experiential basis, because there have been no recognised development routes, although there are now a number of actions that individuals, organisations and training organisations can take and tools that can be used to assess and to develop skills in leading and managing with political awareness (Hartley et al, 2007).

The internal context of the organisation (its structure, culture and history) is also important. The organisational context shapes how formal leadership development programmes are used and also how informal and emergent experiences are drawn on, and how people are selected for such experiences (Alimo-Metcalfe and Lawler, 2001; Hartley and Hinksman, 2003). Leadership development can be considered both in terms of formal programmes (for example, training courses, development programmes, educational programmes) and also in terms of informal activities that support leadership development (for example, on-the-job experiences chosen to create 'stretch' for the participant, mentoring and so on), and different organisations have different preferences for emphasis on each. The organisational context may also influence whether the main focus is on the individual, the team or group, sets of roles (for example, medical directors, aspiring chief executives; fast-track programmes), or concerned with the whole organisation (for example, organisation development). The organisational culture and procedures may also have an impact on who is seen as potential 'leadership material' and who gets access to formal leadership development activities.

Organisational context and conditions (for example, organisational structure, resources, culture, HR strategy) may have an impact on how leadership potential is identified as well as developed (Hartley and Hinksman, 2003). An initial stage of any leadership development programme or set of activities is to identify (and then recruit) individuals or groups for leadership development. There are a number of ways in which this may occur in organisations and this is also often closely related to the (implicit) model of leadership – for example, whether the organisation is making assumptions about strong (single, individual) leadership or distributed leadership. How far down or into the organisation there is a search for leadership potential is a key strategic decision of organisations, although not always recognised as such.

A practical difficulty may be in getting staff released to go on a training programme, either to get the time to go, or to have duties delegated in order to free up the time to go. As organisations become more team-based and decentralised, being away from the office can create pressures for colleagues, leading to reluctance to go away even on short courses in leadership development (see for example, Hartley, 2002a).

The organisational context is often critical in affecting how far there is a transfer of the development learning back into the organisation after the leadership development programme (Day, 2001; McCauley and van Elsor, 2004). Difficulties may arise in identifying how to apply ideas and practices back on the job, or in losing motivation once having left the hothouse of the leadership development programme. Difficulties can also occur in winning the hearts and minds of immediate line managers or more senior managers who have not been part of the leadership development programme (Huczynski and Lewis, 2007), and/or working in an organisational culture that is not conducive to the new approaches (Alimo-Metcalfe and Lawler, 2001).

The challenges of leadership

In Chapter 5, we examined a range of challenges, also called the tasks or purposes of leadership. At a general level, leadership development can be used to help distinguish between adaptive and technical problems (Heifetz, 1994), also called wicked and tame problems (Grint, 2005b). Deciding whether a problem is 'tame' or 'wicked' and therefore whether it requires technical or adaptive leadership is an important skill, with enormous consequences for how the context and purpose is defined, and how the leader works with groups and individuals relevant to solving or addressing the problem. How can leadership development programmes focus on and help leaders to tackle these issues? A focus on problem-identification not just problem-solving is increasingly being thought of as a key skill for leaders and managers (Sparrow, 2000; Gardner, 2004). Interpreting the type of challenge and the ways of leading responses is an important issue for leadership development. Glatter (2008) reinforces this: "Raw experience is not a sufficient guide to learning: leaders may need help in structuring and analysing experience to be able to use it as a resource for learning" (p 6). Interpreting leadership challenges requires conceptual models, but also the flexibility to adapt mental models and mindsets where the changing context requires this.

A further type of challenge relates to leading and managing organisational and cultural change through programmes of improvement and innovation. Such challenges require technical knowledge and skills (for example, lean management, value chain analysis, improvement science), while also needing the skills for the leadership and management of change. Knowing how to influence others to change accepted patterns of thinking and established work practices in the workplace, how to encourage innovation and the management of risk, are important leadership skills. These may be a mix of 'adaptive' and 'technical' challenges. Leadership development in healthcare, therefore, needs to help develop the mental models and skills for change management in healthcare.

Some challenges lie outside as well as inside the organisation. There is more work to be done in understanding the effective leadership of partnerships, of working with local communities and of working with elected politicians. How far are the current leadership development programmes in healthcare addressing these challenges? And what can be passed on from those who have led major challenges (mergers, reconfigurations, turnaround situations) to help those who have not yet faced these testing situations? There is also more work to be done on designing development programmes that develop leadership cadres across the whole public service system (Benington and Hartley, 2009).

One approach to emergent leadership development is through designing stretching job assignments, or through using secondments and other job-based experiences. How far do healthcare organisations capitalise on learning from job challenges by carefully analysing the different kinds of leadership challenge they may represent?

The capabilities of leadership

Leadership development is based on the assumption that capabilities (competencies, qualities, skills, mindsets) can be learned; that they can be acquired rather than given or inherited. There is now considerable evidence from a variety of sources that many leadership qualities can be learned, even for many of those skills where some people have a more natural aptitude than others (Burke and Cooper, 2006).

Many organisations have developed their own leadership capabilities framework, including the NHS and the police service. The models on which these are based will influence the approach to leadership development, including the qualities that are sought in effective leaders and how these are evaluated. Kelloway and Barling (2000), for example, show how focusing on each different dimension of transformational leadership (the four elements of idealised influence, inspirational motivation, intellectual stimulation and individualised consideration) provides different implications for the focus of leadership development.

Some have argued that increasingly there is a need to think of post-transformational leadership development where the focus is less on influencing the immediate individual or group and more on shaping the organisational structure and culture in ways that support particular goals and behaviours and enhance organisational learning (Fullan, 2001; Storey, 2004; Yukl, 2009).

Capability models lie at the heart of many leadership development programmes, with a great emphasis on first defining a skill set (or more widely defined as a mindset) and then designing activities to foster and enhance those skills. However, this book has suggested that there may be dangers in this approach if leadership is not seen in a wider perspective, which includes consideration of context and the challenges of leadership. If there is anything we know about effective leadership, it is that it is dependent on the specific context and challenges. The idea of a universalistic response, based on universal qualities, is not upheld by the evidence.

Consequences of leadership development

If the question about consequences for leadership theory is whether there is evidence that leadership has an impact on organisational performance, then the parallel question for leadership development is: how do we assess whether leadership development makes a difference not just to individuals but also to organisational change and improvement?

Unfortunately, for a number of leadership development approaches, evaluation is still quite rudimentary. Problems range from an inadequate theory of leadership and leadership development such that evaluation is not possible, to inadequate data collection or the wrong type of data collection, to making inappropriate interpretations from the evidence collected. Others argue that politics means that evaluation is risky for the organisation, both because different stakeholders have different priorities and also because of the problems if the evaluation were to reveal substantial weaknesses in a flagship programme of leadership development (Mabey and Finch-Lees, 2008).

In order for evaluation to occur with any degree of robustness, there is a need for a reasonably clear specification of what forms the basis of the leadership development. In other words, what is the model of leadership being used, and how is the development hypothesised to impact on leadership performance and organisational performance?

There is a range of leadership development tools and techniques being used to try to enhance leadership and organisational performance, such as: 360 degree feedback; mentoring; coaching; networking; action learning; job challenges; secondments; formal and educational programmes; fast-track cohorts; organisation development; and partnership working. Some of these are methods of identifying leadership potential as well as means of enhancing leadership for the organisation (Hartley and Hinksman [2003] examine these for the health sector). However, an explicit model of leadership and leadership development is not always articulated and it is sometimes assumed that the initiative by itself is automatically going to improve leadership.

As each method is used, consideration might be given to whether the impacts of leadership development are expected to be planned or emergent, and whether building human or social capital, drawing on Figure 8.2 earlier in this chapter. The quadrants imply different approaches to leadership development and therefore they are likely to require different approaches to evaluation. Where the focus in leadership development is on prescription, then evaluation is able to use a scientific approach, with the clear specification of goals, performance standards, competencies and so on. Where the focus is on emergent properties, then evaluation will need to take a more qualitative and more formative approach, as the outcomes cannot be pre-specified.

The research design for evaluation will also be influenced by whether the focus is on the individual or the social group (team, organisational service unit, whole organisation, critical mass of professionals). Reviews of evaluation approaches in healthcare, commissioned by the NHS Leadership Centre (Williams, 2004a, 2004b), are valuable in setting out possible evaluation approaches and their strengths and weaknesses.

Evaluation of leadership development has both subjective and objective elements. The objective elements may come from organisational performance measures (although these are themselves influenced by human factors such as performance pressure and expectations). The subjective elements come from the perceptions and mental models that individuals and groups hold about leadership and leadership development.

The purpose of the evaluation is also important. Is the key purpose to 'prove' or to 'improve' the leadership development approach? If the former, more rigorous evaluation designs can be important in order to be able to interpret the evidence with reasonable confidence in relation to alternative explanations of the data. If improving the leadership is the goal, then qualitative evidence, based on perceptions and experience as well as hard data, may be important to fine-tune and develop the approach.

The contingent nature of leadership (that it is affected by and affects the contexts, the challenges, the characteristics and the capabilities) means that leadership development is also likely to be contingent, and this suggests searching for leadership development impacts using a realist evaluation perspective (Pawson and Tilley, 1997; Tilley, 2010) based on 'what works, for whom, when, in what circumstances and why' rather than seeking universal principles.

Policy and practice implications:

- Clear thinking about leadership development is essential. Using the analytical framework presented in this book will help to ask critical questions to ensure alignment between strategic purposes and leadership development practices.
- There is no 'one best way' to achieve high-quality leadership development. Clear planning is needed to ensure that leadership development fits with the organisation's strategic direction and priorities, supports appropriate skills and values, is resource-efficient, and contributes not only to individual development but also to organisational change and improvement.
- It is useful to think about how far the emphasis in any particular leadership development approach is focused on planned (for example, formal training and programmes) or emergent (for example, job challenges) features; also whether the focus is on individuals or groups (for example, teams, units, cohorts).
- Planning leadership development needs to cover: how people are selected; the curriculum design; the pedagogical principles; the actual activities; the organisational framework; and how leadership development is evaluated.
- Clarifying the concept of leadership underlying the leadership development is essential, otherwise the approach may be inappropriate for the needs of the organisation. How clear is the organisation about its views of what constitutes effective leadership and what constitutes effective management? For example, if the organisation relies on a 'heroic' concept of individual leadership then it may miss opportunities to develop shared or distributed leadership.
- Thinking about characteristics focuses on the roles that leaders occupy. The sources and resources for influence are important so that the appropriate skills can be developed. Direct leaders may require different skills from indirect leaders. Clinicians need different skills if they are to move from clinical practice to clinical leadership. And, to take another example, shared leadership has implications for the ways in which leadership development may be structured.

- Leadership development that helps leaders to understand and interpret existing contexts and potential future scenarios is important in preparation for leading in a complex and changing world.
- If healthcare benefits from a 'whole-systems' perspective, then leadership development might incorporate that view, with some programmes deliberately linking people across different levels of government and across services and sectors.
- The organisational context has a large impact on the effectiveness of leadership development – who gets selected as leadership material, how transfer of learning back to the workplace happens. Paying attention to pre- and post-leadership development activities is critical.
- More attention could be paid to using job challenges and real-life dilemmas more effectively as an emergent approach to leadership development. These require support for reflection from the experiences.
- The challenges of leadership emphasise the need to distinguish between technical and adaptive (tame and wicked) problems. Using leadership development to enhance not just problem-solving but also problem-identification is increasingly important. Interpreting the type of leadership challenge and the ways of leading responses is an important issue for leadership development.
- The key skills of leadership will be influenced by the capabilities model being used. But capabilities need to be seen in the context of job demands and organisational context. Developing universalistic models of capability may not be helpful.
- Cross-sector leadership development may be particularly important to help develop skills in emotional intelligence and leadership with political awareness.
- It is worth paying attention right at the design stage of leadership development to the potential consequences of leadership. What are the outcomes being sought?
- Organisational outcomes are important but so are the wider outcomes for the public and for the public sphere.
- Designing in evaluation at an early stage will help ensure that leadership development is focused and that it can be modified over time using systematic feedback.

CHAPTER 9

Conclusions

In this book, we have created an analytical framework – the Warwick Six C Leadership Framework – in order to make sense of the 'blooming, buzzing, confusion' in the field of leadership studies. The Six C Framework provides a lens through which to scrutinise the leadership literature, providing questions to explore from different perspectives and marshalling ideas and evidence to inform practice. The book aims both to provide high-quality concepts, ideas and analysis and also to ensure that these are relevant and valuable for those who take practical leadership roles in healthcare, or who are involved in leadership development in this sector.

There are six elements in this analytical framework: the *concepts* that are used to define leadership; the *characteristics* of the roles and resources that have an impact on the types of leadership influence; the *contexts* of leadership in healthcare; the *challenges* of leadership in terms of the purposes or goals of leadership; the *capabilities* of leadership; and the *consequences* of leadership.

This framework is particularly relevant in the dynamic and changing context of the NHS and of healthcare more generally. The book offers a view of leadership beyond the traditional focus on the individual and argues that leadership needs to be seen as grounded in particular social, organisational and inter-organisational contexts and cultures. There is a need to think not only about leaders as individuals but also about leadership constellations, as leadership is often shared across a group of people with different sources of authority, legitimacy and expertise for different aspects of complex challenges.

Our conclusions are brief, because each of the chapters has summarised key aspects of each element of the framework at the beginning of the chapter and provided implications for policy and practice at the end of each chapter.

Each of the elements of the Warwick Six C Framework offers a set of perspectives and ways of examining the evidence and practice in relation to leadership. For example, the concepts element alerts the reader to the idea that different people may use the language and ideas of leadership to mean very different things, for example, focusing on the person, the position or the processes of leadership, and that therefore it can be helpful to be aware of these different meanings, because this will affect the ways in which leadership is understood, practised and developed. Or, to take another example, the challenges element provides ideas and evidence about the purposes of leadership and how these are framed. It is particularly important to 'begin with the end in mind' and to think about 'leadership for what'. It is valuable to think hard about the specific problems that leadership seeks to address, and how to tackle these, recognising that the challenges may be dynamic and that they may sometimes be at least partly constituted, or framed, through the sense-making activities of leadership. The analysis of the specific problem or challenge to be addressed lies at the heart of leadership because the analysis of what healthcare is trying to achieve, both in the long term and the short term, is central to leadership behaviours, processes and actions. If it is to be effective, leadership cannot be divorced from the analysis of the context and the challenges. We will not, here, cover the other four elements but refer the reader to the summaries at the beginning and the implications at the end of each chapter.

There is an implicit seventh 'C' in this framework – which is *connectedness*. Each element of leadership is connected with the other elements, and it would be foolish to focus on one or maybe two elements of the framework without considering the whole inter-connected system. For example, it is not feasible to think about or try to develop the capabilities of leadership without taking into account the leadership model (concepts), the sources of power and legitimacy for leadership (characteristics), the external policy contexts and the internal organisational context (contexts), to think about the goals or purposes for which leadership is exercised (challenges) or to have some awareness of the impacts or possible impacts, both for the task in hand and also to achieve positive outcomes for the public sphere (consequences). The connectedness of the framework is also highly relevant for leadership development, which is why the penultimate chapter uses the Six C Framework to structure the questions and assemble the evidence in relation to the efficacy of leadership development.

The dynamic context of healthcare means that leaders need to pay close and constant attention to the framing of challenges and an assessment of the contexts within which leadership is exercised in the service of healthcare, while also taking into account potential consequences of particular framings and particular actions. Many traditional leadership frameworks have failed to keep pace with a rapidly changing world and this is one of the reasons why the connectedness of the Six C Framework is essential. Leadership itself is a dynamic process of influence not a static set of defined skills to be deployed.

The evidence from leadership studies and experience in healthcare is that there is no 'one best way' of being an effective leader. For example, a direct leader (working face-to-face with their team) will exercise leadership in a different way from an indirect leader (whose leadership may be through design of the organisation or by influencing the overall culture of healthcare at organisational or system levels, and through social marketing or mass communication). A well-respected clinician has a different source of authority from an experienced senior manager – and different again from a local or national politician. Leadership varies by the characteristics of a specific role and resource base. Or leadership may vary by the challenge to be addressed – a 'technical', tame problem calls for different leadership than an 'adaptive', wicked problem. Yet again, the different phases of a complex change, such as a merger or a substantial change in strategy, may call for different leadership styles, for example transformational and transactional leadership will each be relevant at different periods in a merger. This takes us back to the critical importance of accurately 'reading' the context in which leadership is exercised. Leadership benefits from an approach that is not uniform or universalistic, but that asks key questions: *what will work, in what circumstances, why and how?* This involves the leader using not a standardised recipe for success (as some leadership books simplistically offer), but rather a conceptual framework that guides the kinds of questions that need to be asked and answered (even if fuzzily or provisionally) in order to be effective. What do we think the problem is here? How is the political, economic and social context influencing the dynamics of this problem? How do other stakeholders see this problem? What interests do they have in this situation? How is the problem changing? What resources can I draw on? Should I focus on being the main leader or can I draw others in to the task? What might be the beneficial and detrimental consequences of particular leadership strategies and actions? We trust that the Six C Framework will help leaders with such questions and that this will inform improved practice in healthcare.

Leadership is constituted not simply as a function of circumstance. While particular problem situations might suggest the value of certain styles or leadership behaviours at certain points, this cannot be simply read off from context. Leaders have a major role in constructing the context not just responding to it. A key theme in this book is about the role of leadership in 'big picture sense-making' and in helping others to understand the context and the challenges ahead. Whether this is through creating a mission or a vision, or by helping others with their own sense-making or sense-breaking, leadership has an important role not only in responding to circumstances, but also in making them. This will be important not only for leading teams, but also for organisational design and organisation development, for working in partnerships and inter-organisational networks, and for shaping the debates about healthcare in the future, with all its myriad challenges.

References

Aarons, G.A. (2006) 'Transformational and transactional leadership: association with attitudes toward evidence-based practice', *Psychiatric Services*, 57 (8), 1162–9.

Albury, D. (2005) 'Fostering innovation in public services', *Public Money and Management*, 25, January, 51–6.

Alexander, J., Comfort, M., Weiner, B. and Bogue, R. (2001) 'Leadership in collaborative community health partnerships', *Nonprofit Management and Leadership*, 12 (2), 159–75.

Alford, J. (2009) *Engaging public sector clients: From service delivery to co-production*, Basingstoke: Palgrave Macmillan.

Alford, J. and O'Flynn, J. (2009) 'Making sense of public value: concepts, critiques and emergent meanings', *International Journal of Public Administration*, 32, 171–91.

Alimo-Metcalfe, B. (1999) 'An investigation of female and male constructs of leadership and empowerment', *Women in Management Review*, 10 (2), 3–8.

Alimo-Metcalfe, B. and Alban-Metcalfe, J. (2002) 'Leadership', in P. Warr (ed) *Psychology at work*, Harmondsworth: Penguin.

Alimo-Metcalfe, B. and Alban-Metcalfe, J. (2004) 'Leadership in public sector organizations', in J. Storey (ed) *Leadership in organizations: Current issues and key trends*, London: Routledge.

Alimo-Metcalfe, B. and Alban-Metcalfe, J. (2005) 'Leadership: time for a new direction?', *Leadership*, 1 (1), 51–71.

Alimo-Metcalfe, B. and Lawler, J. (2001) 'Leadership development in UK companies at the beginning of the twenty-first century: lessons for the NHS?', *Journal of Management in Medicine*, 15 (5), 387–404.

Arnold, K., Turner, N., Barling, J., Kelloway, K. and McKee, M. (2007) 'Transformational leadership and psychological well-being: the mediating role of meaningful work', *Journal of Occupational Health Psychology*, 12 (3), 193–203.

Avolio, B. (1999) *Full leadership development*, Thousand Oaks, CA: Sage.

Avolio, B., Bass, B. and Jung, D. (1990) 'Re-examining the components of transformational and transactional leadership using the multifactor leadership questionnaire', *Journal of Occupational and Organizational Psychology*, 72 (4), 441–62.

Avolio, B.J., Zhu, W.C. and Bhatia, P. (2004) 'Transformational leadership and organizational commitment: mediating role of psychological empowerment and moderating role of structural distance', *Journal of Organizational Behaviour*, 25 (8), 951–68.

Bailey, C. and Burr, J. (2005) *Luck, legacy or leadership: The contribution of leadership to sustained organisational success in NHS Trusts*, London: The NHS Leadership Centre and Cranfield School of Management.

Barling, J., Turner, N., Kelloway, K., Sivanathan, N., Arnold, K. and Louglin, C. (2009) 'Transformational leadership and employee well-being', Working paper, Kingston, Ontario: Queen's University.

Barrett, L., Plotnikoff, R.C., Raine, K. and Anderson, D. (2005) 'Development of measures of organizational leadership for health promotion', *Health Education and Behaviour*, 32 (2), 195–207.

Bass, B. (1985) *Leadership and performance beyond expectations*, New York: Free Press.

Bass, B. (1998) *Transformational leadership*, Mahwah, NJ: Lawrence Erlbaum.

Bass, B. (1999) 'Two decades of research and development in transformational leadership', *European Journal of Work and Organizational Psychology*, 12, 47–59.

Bass, B. and Avolio, B. (1990) 'The implications of transactional and transformational leadership for individual, team and organizational development', *Research in Organizational Change and Development*, 4, 231–72.

Bate, P. and Robert, G. (2002) 'Knowledge management and communities of practice in the private sector: lessons for modernizing the National Health Service in England and Wales', *Public Administration*, 80 (4), 643–63.

Bate, P. and Robert, G. (2007) 'Toward more user-centric OD', *Journal of Applied Behavioral Science*, 43, 41–66.

Benington, J. (2000) 'The modernization and improvement of government and public services', *Public Money and Management*, April–June, 3–8.

Benington, J. (2001) 'Partnership as networked governance? Legitimation, innovation, problem-solving and co-ordination', in M. Geddes and J. Benington (eds) *Local partnerships and social exclusion in the European Union*, London: Routledge.

Benington, J. (2004) *Public sector leadership and management development in Wales*, Coventry: Institute of Governance and Public Management, University of Warwick.

Benington, J. (2006) *Reforming public services*, Sunningdale: National School of Government.

Benington, J. (2010) 'From private choice to public value', in J. Benington and J. Moore (eds) *Public value: Theory and practice*, Basingstoke: Palgrave Macmillan.

Benington, J. and Hartley, J. (2009) *Whole systems go! Leadership across the whole public service system*, London: National School of Government.

Benington, J. and Moore, J. (2010) *Public value: Theory and practice*, Basingstoke: Palgrave Macmillan.

Benington, J. and Turbitt, I. (2007) 'Adaptive leadership and the policing of Drumcree demonstrations in Northern Ireland', *Leadership*, 3 (4), 371–95.

Benington, J., Hartley, J., Neilsen, R. and Notten, T. (2008) 'Innovation, design and delivery of MPA programmes for public leaders and managers in Europe', *International Journal of Public Sector Management*, 21 (4), 383–99.

Bennis, W. (1999) 'Exemplary leadership is impossible without full inclusion, initiatives and co-operation of followers', *Organizational Dynamics*, 28, 71–9.

Bennis, W. and Nanus, B. (1985) *Leaders: The strategies for taking charge*, New York: Harper and Row.

Bennis, W. and Thomas, R. (2002) *Geeks and geezers: How era, values and defining moments shape leaders*, Boston, MA: Harvard Business School Press.

Bennis, W., Spreitzer, G. and Cummings, T.G. (2001) *The future of leadership*, San Francisco, CA: Jossey Bass.

Berwick, D. (1994) 'Eleven worthy aims for clinical leadership of health system reform', *Journal of the American Medical Association*, 272 (10), 797–802.

Bion, W. (1961) *Experiences in groups*, London: Tavistock.

Blackler, F. (2006) 'Chief executives and the modernisation of the English National Health Service', *Leadership*, 2 (1), 5–30.

Blackler, F. and Kennedy, A. (2004) 'The design and evaluation of a leadership programme for experienced chief executives from the public sector', *Management Learning*, 35 (2), 181–203.

Bolden, R. and Gosling, J. (2006) 'Leadership competencies: time to change the tune?', *Leadership*, 2 (2), 147–63.

Bolden, R., Wood, M. and Gosling, J. (2006) 'Is the NHS leadership qualities framework missing the wood for the trees?', in A. Casebeer, A. Harrison and A. Mark (eds) *Innovations in health care: A reality check*, New York: Palgrave.

Borrill, C., West, M. and Dawson, J. (2003) 'The relationship between leadership, people management, staff satisfaction and intentions to leave', Report, Birmingham: Aston Business School.

Boyatzis, R. (1982) *The competent manager: A model for effective performance*, New York: Wiley.

Boyatzis, R. (2006) 'Leadership competencies', in R. Burke and C.L. Cooper (eds) *Inspiring leaders*, London: Routledge, pp 119–31.

Boyne, G. (2004) 'A 3 Rs strategy for public service turnaround: retrenchment, repositioning and reorganization', *Public Money and Management*, 24 (2), 97–103.

Boyne, G. (2008) 'Public service failure and turnaround: towards a contingency model', in J. Hartley, C. Donaldson, C. Skelcher and M. Wallace (2008) *Managing to improve public services*, Cambridge: Cambridge University Press.

Brazier, D. (2005) 'Influence of contextual factors on health-care leadership', *Leadership and Organization Development Journal*, 26 (1/2), 128–40.

Briscoe, J. and Hall, D. (1999) 'An alternative approach and new guidelines', *Organizational Dynamics*, 28 (2), 37–52.

Bryman, A. (1992) *Charisma and leadership in organizations*, London: Sage.

Buchanan, D. (2003) 'Effective organizations and leadership development: trends and issues', Report commissioned for the NHS Leadership Centre, Leicester: Leicester Business School.

Buchanan, D., Fitzgerald, L. and Ketley, D. (2007) *The sustainability and spread of organizational change*, London: Routledge.

Burdett Trust for Nursing (2006) *An exploratory study of the clinical content of NHS trust board meetings, in an attempt to identify good practice*, London: Burdett Trust for Nursing.

Burgoyne, J., Pedler, M. and Boydell, T. (2005) *Leadership development: Current practice, future perspectives*, London: Corporate Research Forum.

Burke, R. (2006a) 'Inspiring leaders: an introduction', in R. Burke and C.L. Cooper (eds) *Inspiring leaders*, London: Routledge, pp 1–30.

Burke, R. (2006b) 'Why leaders fail: exploring the dark side', in R. Burke and C.L. Cooper (eds) *Inspiring leaders*, London: Routledge.

Burke, R. and Cooper, C.L. (2006) *Inspiring leaders*, London: Routledge.

Burnes, B. (2004) *Managing change* (4th edn), London: Pitman.

Burns, J. (1978) *Leadership*, New York: Harper and Row.

Burns, T. and Stalker, G. (1994) *The management of innovation* (3rd edn), Oxford: Oxford University Press.

Bynner, W. (1944) *The way of life according to Lao Tzu*, New York: Putnam.

Cabinet Office (2001) *Strengthening leadership in the public sector*, London: Cabinet Office.

Cha, S. and Edmondson, A. (2006) 'When values backfire: leadership, attribution and disenchantment in a values-driven organization', *Leadership Quarterly*, 17 (1), 57–78.

Cherniss, C. (2006) 'Leadership and emotional intelligence', in R. Burke and C.L. Cooper (eds) *Inspiring leaders*, London: Routledge.

Clark, J., Spurgeon, P. and Hamilton, P. (2008) 'Medical professionalism: leadership competency – an essential ingredient', *International Journal of Clinical Leadership*, 16 (1), 3–9.

Coleman, A. and Glendinning, C. (2004) 'Local authority scrutiny of health: making the views of the community count?', *Health Expectations*, 7 (1), 29–39.

Collinson, D. (2006) 'Rethinking followership: a post-structuralist analysis of follower identities', *The Leadership Quarterly*, 17 (2), 172–89.

Conger, J. and Kanungo, R. (1987) 'Toward a behavioral theory of charismatic leadership in organizational settings', *Academy of Management Review*, 12, 637–47.

Corrigan, P., Lickey, S., Campion, J. and Rashid, F. (2000) 'Mental health team leadership and consumers' satisfaction and quality of life', *Psychiatric Services*, 51 (6), 781–5.

Corrigan, P., Diwan, S., Campion, J. and Rashid, F. (2002) 'Transformational leadership and the mental health team', *Administration and Policy in Mental Health*, 30 (2), 97–108.

Day, D. (2001) 'Leadership development: a review in context', *Leadership Quarterly*, 11, 581–613.

Denis, J.-L., Langley, A. and Cazale, L. (1996) 'Leadership and strategic change under ambiguity', *Organization Studies*, 17 (4), 673–99.

Denis, J.-L., Lamothe, L. and Langley, A. (2001) 'The dynamics of collective leadership and strategic change in pluralistic organizations', *Academy of Management Journal*, 44 (4), 809–37.

Denis, J.-L., Langley, A. and Rouleau, L. (2005) 'Rethinking leadership in public organizations', in E. Ferlie, L. Lynn and C. Pollitt (eds) *The Oxford handbook of public management*, Oxford: Oxford University Press.

Denis, J.-L., Langley, A. and Rouleau, L. (forthcoming) 'The practice of leadership in the messy world of organizations', *Leadership*.

DH (Department of Health) (2000) *The NHS plan: A plan for investment, a plan for reform*, London: The Stationery Office.

DH (2008) *Next stage review: High quality care for all*, London: Department of Health.

Dickinson, H. (2009) 'The outcomes of health and social care partnerships', in J. Glasby and H. Dickinson (eds) *International perspectives on health and social care: Partnership working in action*, Chichester: Wiley-Blackwell.

Dickinson, H. and Ham, C. (2008) *Engaging doctors in leadership: Review of the literature*, Birmingham: University of Birmingham.

Dickinson, H., Peck, E. and Smith, J. (2006) 'Leadership in organisational transition – what can we learn from research evidence?', Report, University of Birmingham.

Dopson, S., Fitzgerald, L. and Gabbay, J. (2005) *Knowledge to action? Evidence-based health care in context*, Oxford: Oxford University Press.

Dulewicz, C., Young, M. and Dulewicz, V. (2005) 'The relevance of emotional intelligence for leadership performance', *Journal of General Management*, 30 (3), 71–86.

Dulewicz, V. and Higgs, M. (2004) 'Can emotional intelligence be developed?', *International Journal of Human Resource Management*, 15, 95–111.

Dunham-Taylor, J. (2000) 'Nurse executive transformational leadership found in participative organizations', *Journal of Nursing Administration*, 30 (5), 241–50.

Dunphy, D. and Stace, D. (1993) 'The strategic management of corporate change', *Human Relations*, 46 (8), 905–18.

DuPree, M. (1998) 'What is leadership?', in G. Hickman (ed) *Leading organizations: Perspectives for a new era*, Thousand Oaks, CA: Sage.

Eagly, A., Johannesen-Schmidt, M. and van Engen, M. (2003) 'Tranformational, transactional and laissez-faire leadership styles: a meta-analysis comparing women and men', *Psychological Bulletin*, 95, 569–91.

Edmondson, A.C. (2004) 'Learning from failure in health care: frequent opportunities, pervasive barriers', *Quality and Safety in Health Care*, 13, 3–9.

Edmonstone, J. and Western, J. (2002) 'Leadership development in healthcare: what do we know?', *Journal of Health Organization and Management*, 16 (1), 34–47.

Endacott, R., Sheaff, R., Jones, R. and Woodward, V. (2008) 'Clinical focus at Board level in English NHS Trusts', Conference paper, European Health Management Association Conference, Athens, June.

Eriksen, E.O. (2001) 'Leadership in a communicative perspective', *Acta Sociologica*, 44 (1), 21–35.

Ferlie, F. and Pettigrew, A. (1996) 'Managing through networks: some issues and implications for the NHS', *British Journal of Management*, 7, S81–S99.

Ferlie, E. and Shortell, S. (2001) 'Improving the quality of health care in the United Kingdom and the United States: a framework for change', *Milbank Quarterly*, 79 (2), 281–315.

Fiedler, F. (1967) *A theory of leadership effectiveness*, New York: McGraw-Hill.

Fleishman, E., Harris, E. and Burtt, H. (1955) *Leadership and supervision in industry*, Research monograph 33, Columbus, OH: Ohio State University, Bureau of Education Research.

Fletcher, C. (2004) 'A review of competency frameworks and core capabilities', in J. Benington (ed) *Report for the Commission on Public Sector Leadership Development in Wales*, Coventry: University of Warwick.

Fletcher, C. (2008) *Appraisal, feedback and development: Making performance review work* (4th edn), London: Routledge.

Flyberg, B. (2001) *Making social science matter*, Cambridge: Cambridge University Press.

Ford, J. (2005) 'Examining leadership through critical feminist readings', *Journal of Health Organization and Management*, 19 (3), 236–51.

French, J. and Raven, B. (1959) 'The bases of social power', in D. Cartwright (ed) *Studies of social power*, Ann Arbor, MI: Institute for Social Research.

Fullan, M. (2001) *Leading in a culture of change*, San Franscisco, CA: Jossey Bass.

Gardner, H. (2004) *Changing minds*, Boston, MA: Harvard Business School Press.

Garman, A.N., Davis-Lenane, D. and Corrigan, P. (2003) 'Factor structure of the transformational leadership model in human service teams', *Journal of Organizational Behaviour*, 24 (6), 803–12.

Gelinas, L.S. and Manthey, M. (1997) 'The impact of organizational redesign on nurse executive leadership', *Journal of Nursing Administration*, 27 (10), 35–42.

Glasby, J. and Dickinson, H. (eds) (2009) *International perspectives on health and social care: Partnership working in action*, Oxford: Blackwell-Wiley.

Glatter, R. (1997) 'Context and capability in educational management', *Educational Management Administration and Leadership*, 25 (2), 181–92.

Glatter, R. (2004) 'Leadership and leadership development in education', in J. Storey (ed) *Leadership in organizations: Current issues and key trends*, London: Routledge.

Glatter, R. (2008) 'Of leadership, management and wisdom. A brief synthesis of selected reports and documents on leadership development', Report, Nottingham: National College for School Leadership.

Gold, J., Thorpe, R. and Mumford, A. (2010) *Gower handbook of leadership and management development*, Farnham: Gower.

Goleman, D. (1995) *Emotional intelligence: Why it can matter more than IQ*, New York: Bantam.

Goleman, D., Boyatzis, R. and McKee, A. (2002) *Primal leadership: Learning to lead with emotional intelligence*, Boston, MA: Harvard Business School Press.

Goodall, A. (2009) *Socrates in the boardroom: Why research universities should be led by top scholars*, Princeton, NJ: Princeton University Press.

Goodwin, N. (1998) 'Leadership in the UK NHS: where are we now?', *Journal of Management in Medicine*, 12 (1), 21–32.

Goodwin, N. (2000) 'Leadership and the UK health service', *Health Policy*, 51 (1), 49–60.

Goodwin, N. (2006) *Leadership in health care: A European perspective*, London: Routledge.

Greenwood, R. and Hinings, R. (1996) 'Understanding radical change: bringing together the old and the new institutionalism', *Academy of Management Review*, 21 (4), 1022–53.

Grint, K. (2000) *The arts of leadership*, Oxford: Oxford University Press.

Grint, K. (2005a) *Leadership: Limits and possibilities*, Basingstoke: Palgrave Macmillan.

Grint, K. (2005b) 'Problems, problems, problems: the social construction of "leadership"', *Human Relations*, 58, 1467–94.

Gronn, P. (2002) 'Distributed leadership as a unit of analysis', *Leadership Quarterly*, 13 (4), 423–51.

Gronn, P. (2009) 'Leadership configurations', *Leadership*, 5 (3), 1–13.

Guo, K. (2004) 'Leadership processes for re-engineering changes to the health care industry', *Journal of Health Organization and Management*, 18 (6), 435–46.

Hackett, M. and Spurgeon, P. (1996) 'Leadership and vision in the NHS: how do we create the "vision thing"', *Health Manpower Management*, 22 (1), 5–9.

Hackett, M. and Spurgeon, P. (1998) 'Developing our leaders in the future', *Health Manpower Management*, 24, 170–77.

Halpin, A. and Winer, B. (1957) 'A factorial study of the leader behavior descriptions', in R. Stogdill and A. Coons (eds) *Leader behavior: Its description and measurement*, Columbus, OH: Bureau of Business Research, Ohio State University.

Ham, C. (2003) 'Improving the performance of health services: the role of clinical leadership', *The Lancet*, 361 (9373), 1978–80.

Ham, C. (2008) 'Doctors in leadership: learning from international experience', *International Journal of Clinical Leadership*, 16 (1), 11–16.

Hartley, J. (2000) 'Leading and managing the uncertainty of strategic change', in P. Flood, S. Carroll, L. Gorman and T. Dromgoole (eds) *Managing strategic implementation*, Oxford: Blackwell, pp 109–22.

Hartley, J. (2002a) 'Leading communities: capabilities and cultures', *Leadership and Organizational Development Journal*, 23, 419–29.

Hartley, J. (2002b) 'Organizational change and development', in P. Warr (ed) *Psychology at work* (5th edn), Harmondsworth: Penguin, pp 399–425.

Hartley, J. (2005) 'Innovation in governance and public services: past and present', *Public Money and Management*, 25, January, 27–34.

Hartley, J. (2008) 'The innovation landscape for public service organizations', in J. Hartley, C. Donaldson, C. Skelcher and M. Wallace (eds) *Managing to improve public services*, Cambridge: Cambridge University Press, pp 195–214.

Hartley, J. (2010a) 'Public sector leadership and management development', in J. Gold, R. Thorpe and A. Mumford (eds) *Gower handbook of leadership and management development*, Aldershot: Gower.

Hartley, J. (2010b) 'Political leadership', in S. Brookes and K. Grint (eds) *The public leadership challenge*, London: Palgrave.

Hartley, J. (2010c) 'Public value through innovation and improvement', in J. Benington and M. Moore (eds) *Public value: Theory and practice*, Basingstoke: Palgrave.

Hartley, J. and Allison, M. (2000) 'The role of leadership in modernisation and improvement of public service', *Public Money and Management*, 20 (2), 35–40.

Hartley, J. and Fletcher, C. (2008) 'Leadership with political awareness: leadership across diverse interests inside and outside the organization', in K. James and J. Collins (eds) *Leadership perspectives: Knowledge into action*, London: Palgrave, pp 157–70.

Hartley, J. and Hinksman, B. (2003) *Leadership development: A systematic review of the literature*, Report, London: NHS Leadership Centre.

Hartley, J. and Rashman, L. (2007) 'How is knowledge transferred between organizations involved in change?', in M. Wallace, M. Fertig and E. Schneller (eds) *Managing change in the public services*, Oxford: Blackwell, pp 173–92.

Hartley, J., Fletcher, C., Wilton, P., Woodman, P. and Ungemach, C. (2007) *Leading with political awareness*, London: Chartered Management Institute.

Hatch, M.J. (1997) *Organization theory: Modern, symbolic and postmodern perspectives*, Oxford: Oxford University Press.

Heifetz, R. (1994) *Leadership without easy answers*, Cambridge, MA: Harvard University Press.

Heifetz, R.A. (2004) 'Adaptive work', in G. Goethals, G. Sorenson and J.M. Burns (eds) *Encyclopedia of leadership*, Thousand Oaks, CA: Sage.

Heifetz, R.A. and Laurie, D.L. (1997) 'The work of leadership', *Harvard Business Review*, 75 (1), 124–34.

Heifetz, R., Grashow, A. and Linsky, M. (2009) 'Leadership in a (permanent) crisis', *Harvard Business Review*, July–August, 62–9.

Henochowicz, S. and Hetherington, D. (2006) 'Leadership coaching in health care', *Leadership and Organization Development Journal*, 27 (3), 183–9.

Hirsch, W. and Strebler, M. (1995) 'Defining managerial skills and competencies', in A. Mumford (ed) *Handbook of Management Development*, Aldershot: Gower.

Hirschhorn, L. (1997) *Reworking authority: Leading and following in the post-modern organization*, Cambridge, MA: MIT Press.

Hoggett, P. (2006) 'Conflict, ambivalence and the contested purpose of public organizations', *Human Relations*, 59 (2), 175–94.

Hollenbeck, G., McCall, M. and Silzer, R. (2009) 'Leadership competency models', in J. Billsberry (ed) *Discovering leadership*, Basingstoke: Palgrave Macmillan.

House, R. and Dessler, G. (1974) 'The path-goal theory of leadership: some post hoc and a priori tests', in J.G. Hunt and L. Larson (eds) *Contingency approaches to leadership*, Carbondale, IL: Southern Illinois University Press.

Huczynski, A. and Lewis, W. (2007) 'An empirical study into the learning transfer process in management training', *Journal of Management Studies*, 17 (2), 227–40.

Huff, A.S. and Moeslein, K. (2004) 'An agenda for understanding leadership in corporate leadership systems', in C. Cooper (ed) *Leadership and management in the 21st century: Business challenges of the future*, Oxford: Oxford University Press, pp 248–70.

Hunt, J. (1991) *Leadership: A new synthesis*, Newbury Park, CA: Sage.

Huxham, C. and Vangen, S. (2000) 'Leadership in the shaping and implementation of collaboration agendas: how things happen in a (not quite) joined-up world', *Academy of Management Journal*, 43 (6), 1159–75.

Iles, P. and Sutherland, V. (2001) *Organizational change: A review for health care managers, professionals and researchers*, London: National Coordinating Centre for Service Delivery and Organization (NCCSDO).

Isaksen, S. and Tidd, J. (2006) *Meeting the innovation challenge: Leadership for transformation and growth*, Chichester: Wiley.

Jackson, B. and Parry, K. (2008) *A very short, fairly interesting and reasonably cheap book about studying leadership*, London: Sage.

Jackson, S. (2000) 'A qualitative evaluation of shared leadership barriers, drivers and recommendations', *Journal of Management in Medicine*, 14 (3/4), 166–78.

Jas, P. and Skelcher, C. (2005) 'Performance decline and turnaround: a theoretical and empirical analysis', *British Journal of Management*, 16 (3), 195–210.

Kan, M.M. and Parry, K.W. (2004) 'Identifying paradox: a grounded theory of leadership in overcoming resistance to change', *Leadership Quarterly*, 15 (4), 467–91.

Kaplan, R. (2006) 'Lopsideness in leaders: strategies for assessing it and correcting it', in R. Burke and C.L. Cooper (eds) *Inspiring leaders*, London: Routledge.

Kaplan, R. and Norton, D. (1996) 'Using the balanced scorecard as a strategic management system', *Harvard Business Review*, 74 (1), 75–85.

Kelloway, E. and Barling, J. (2000) 'What have we learned about developing transformational leaders', *Leadership and Organization Development Journal*, 21, 355–62.

Kelloway, K., Sivanathan, N., Francis, L. and Barling, J. (2005) 'Poor leadership', in J. Barling, E.K. Kelloway and M. Frone (eds) *Handbook of work stress*, Thousand Oaks, CA: Sage Publications.

Kets de Vries M (2006) *The leader on the couch: A clinical approach to changing people and organizations*, Chichester: Wiley.

Kimberly, J. and de Pouvourville, G. (1993) *The migration of managerial innovation: Diagnosis related groups and healthcare*, San Francisco, CA: Jossey Bass.

Kotter, J. (1990) *What leaders really do*, Boston, MA: Harvard Business School Press.

Kouzes, J. and Posner, B. (1995) *The leadership challenge* (4th edn), San Francisco, CA: Jossey Bass.

Laschinger, H., Wong, C., McMahon, L. and Kaufman, C. (1999) 'Leader behaviour impact on staff nurse empowerment, job tension and work effectiveness', *Journal of Nursing Administration*, 29 (5), 28–39.

Lasker, R., Weiss, E. and Miller, R. (2001) 'Partnership synergy: a practical framework for studying and strengthening the collaborative advantage', *Milbank Quarterly*, 79 (2), 179–205.

Leach, L.S. (2005) 'Nurse executive transformational leadership and organizational commitment', *Journal of Nursing Administration*, 35 (5), 228–37.

Leach, S. and Wilson, D. (2000) *Local political leadership*, Bristol: The Policy Press.

Leach, S. and Wilson, D. (2002) 'Rethinking local political leadership', *Public Administration*, 80 (4), 665–89.

Leach, S., Hartley, J., Lowndes, V., Wilson, D. and Downe, J. (2005) *Local political leadership in England and Wales*, York: The Joseph Rowntree Foundation.

Locke, E. (1991) *The essence of leadership*, New York: Lexington Books.

Locock, L., Dopson, S., Chambers, D. and Gabbay, J. (2001) 'Understanding the role of opinion leaders in improving clinical effectiveness', *Social Science and Medicine*, 53 (6), 745–57.

Lord, R., DeVader, C. and Allinger, G. (1986) 'A meta-analysis of the relation between personality traits and leadership perceptions: an application of validity generalization procedures', *Journal of Applied Psychology*, 71, 402–10.

Mabey, C. and Finch-Lees, T. (2008) *Management and leadership development*, London: Sage.

Mannion, R., Davies, H. and Marshall, M. (2005) 'Cultural characteristics of "high" and "low" performing hospitals', *Journal of Health Organization and Management*, 19 (6), 431–9.

Manojilovich, M. (2005) 'The effect of nursing leadership on hospital nurses' professional practice behaviors', *Journal of Nursing Administration*, 35 (7/8), 366–74.

Marion, R. and Uhl-Bien, M. (2001) 'Leadership of complex organizations', *Leadership Quarterly*, 12 (4), 389–418.

Marley, K., Collier, D. and Goldstein, S. (2004) 'The role of clinical and process quality in achieving patient satisfaction in hospitals', *Decision Sciences*, 35 (3), 349–69.

Marnoch, G., McKee, L. and Dinnie, N. (2000) 'Between organizations and institutions: legitimacy and medical managers', *Public Administration*, 78, 967–87.

Marquand, D. (2004) *The decline of the public*, Cambridge: Polity Press.

Marsh, D. and Stoker, G. (2002) *Theory and methods in political science* Basingstoke: Palgrave Macmillan.

Martinko, M., Harvey, P. and Douglas, S. (2007) 'The role, function and contribution of attribution theory to leadership: a review', *Leadership Quarterly*, 18 (6), 561–85.

Marturano, A. and Gosling, J. (2008) *Leadership: The key concepts*, London: Routledge.

Matthews, G., Zeinder, M. and Roberts, D. (2002) *Emotional intelligence: Science and myth*, Cambridge, MA: MIT Press.

Mayer, J. and Salovey, P. (1993) 'The intelligence of emotional intelligence', *Intelligence*, 17, 433–42.

McCauley, C. and van Elsor, E. (2004) 'The Center for Creative Leadership handbook of leadership development', San Franscisco, CA: Jossey Bass.

McDaniel, R. (1997) 'Strategic leadership: a view from quantum and chaos theories', *Health Care Management Review*, 22 (1), 21–31.

McDonagh, K.J. (2006) 'Hospital governing boards: a study of their effectiveness in relation to organizational performance', *Journal of Healthcare Management*, 51 (6), 377–89.

McNulty, T. and Ferlie, E. (2004) *Reengineering health care: The complexities of organizational transformation*, Oxford: Oxford University Press.

Meindl, J. and Ehrlich, S. (1987) 'The romance of leadership and the evaluation of organizational performance', *Academy of Management Journal*, 30 (1), 91–109.

Menzies Lyth, I. (1988) 'The functioning of social systems as a defence against anxiety', in I. Menzies Lyth, *Containing anxiety in institutions: Selected essays, Vol. 1*, London: Free Association Books, pp 43–85.

Millward, L. and Bryan, K. (2005) 'Clinical leadership in healthcare: a position statement', *Leadership in Health Services*, 18 (2), 13–25.

Mintzberg, H. (1973) *The nature of managerial work*, New York: Harper and Row.

Mintzberg, H. (1978) 'Patterns in strategy formation', *Management Science*, 24 (9), 934–48.

Mole, G. (2004) 'Can leadership be taught?', in J. Storey (ed) *Leadership in organizations: Current issues and key trends*, London: Routledge.

Moore, M. (1995) *Creating public value*, Cambridge, MA: Harvard University Press.

Morgan, G. (1997) *Images of organization*, London: Sage.

Morrell, K. and Hartley, J. (2006) 'A model of political leadership', *Human Relations*, 59 (4), 483–504.

Morrison, R.S., Jones, L. and Fuller, B. (1997) 'The relation between leadership style and empowerment on job satisfaction of nurses', *Journal of Nursing Administration*, 27 (5), 27–34.

Moses, J. and Knutsen, T. (2007) *Ways of knowing*, Basingstoke: Palgrave Macmillan.

Munshi, N., Oke, A., Puranam, P., Stafylarakis, M., Towells, S., Moeslein, K. and Neely, A. (2005) *Leadership for innovation*, London: Advanced Institute for Management Research.

Nadler, D. and Tushman, M. (1980) 'A model for diagnosing organizational behaviour', *Organizational Dynamics*, 9, 35–51.

Nadler, D. and Tushman, M. (1990) 'Beyond the charismatic leader: leadership and organizational change', *California Management Review*, 32, 77–97.

Neath, A. (2007) 'Layers of leadership: hidden influencers of healthcare', in D. Buchanan, L. Fitzgerald and D. Ketley (eds) *The sustainability and spread of organisational change*, London: Routledge.

NHS (2005) 'NHS Leadership Qualities Framework', available at: www. NHSLeadershipQualities.nhs.uk (accessed 24 August 2009).

Nielson, K., Randall, R., Yarker, J. and Brenner, S. (2008) 'The effects of transformational change on followers' perceived work characteristics and psychological well-being: a longitudinal study', *Work and Stress*, 22, 16–32.

O'Connor, P. and Day, D. (2007) 'Shifting the emphasis of leadership development: from "me" to "all of us"', in J. Conger and R. Riggio (eds) *The practice of leadership*, San Francisco, CA: Jossey Bass.

Osborn, R., Hunt, J.G. and Jauch, L. (2002) 'Toward a contextual theory of leadership', *Leadership Quarterly*, 13 (6), 797–837.

Osborne, S. and Brown, K. (2005) *Managing change and innovation in public service organizations*, London: Routledge.

Øvretveit, J. (2005a) 'Leading improvement', *Journal of Health Organization and Management*, 19 (6), 413–30.

Øvretveit, J. (2005b) *The leaders' role in quality and safety improvement: A review of research and guidance*, Stockholm: Karolinska Institute.

Parry, K. and Bryman, A. (2006) 'Leadership in organizations', in S. Clegg, C. Hardy, T. Lawrence and W. Nord (eds) *The Sage handbook of organization studies*, London: Sage.

Pawson, R. and Tilley, N. (1997) *Realistic evaluation*, London: Sage.

Peck, E. and Dickinson, H. (2008) *Managing and leading in inter-agency settings*, Bristol: The Policy Press.

Peck, E., Dickinson, H. and Smith, J. (2006) 'Transforming or transacting? The role of leaders in organisational transition', *British Journal of Leadership in Public Services*, 2 (3), 4–14.

Pfeffer, J. (1981) 'Management as symbolic action', *Research in Organizational Behavior*, 3, 1–52.

PIU (Performance and Innovation Unit) (2000) *Strengthening leadership in the public sector*, London: Cabinet Office.

Porter, L. and McLaughlin, G. (2006) 'Leadership and the organizational context: like the weather?', *Leadership Quarterly*, 17, 559–76.

Pye, A. (2005) 'Leadership and organizing: sensemaking in action', *Leadership*, 1 (1), 31–49.

Rashman, L. and Hartley, J. (2002) 'Leading and learning? Knowledge transfer in the Beacon Council Scheme', *Public Administration*, 80, 523–42.

Ray, T., Clegg, S. and Gordon, R. (2004) 'A new look at dispersed leadership: power, knowledge and context', in J. Storey (ed) *Leadership in organizations: Current issues and key trends*, London: Routledge.

Reyatt, K. (2008) 'Strategic visioning', in A. Marturano and J. Gosling (eds) *Leadership: The key concepts*, London: Routledge.

Rittel, H. and Webber, M. (1973) 'Dilemmas in a general theory of planning', *Policy Sciences*, 4, 155–69.

Rodgers, H., Gold, J., Frearson, M. and Holden, R. (2003) 'The rush to leadership: explaining leadership development in the public sector', Working paper, Leeds: Leeds Business School.

Rost, J. (1998) 'Leadership and management', in G. Hickman (ed) *Leading organizations: Perspectives for a new era*, Thousand Oaks, CA: Sage.

Rousseau, D. (2006) 'Is there such a thing as evidence-based management', *Academy of Management Review*, 31 (2), 256–69.

Ryde, R. (2007) *Thought leadership: Moving hearts and minds*, Basingstoke: Palgrave Macmillan.

Salaroo, M. and Burnes, B. (1998) 'The impact of a market system on the public sector: a study of organizational change in the NHS', *International Journal of Public Sector Management*, 11 (6), 451–67.

Schein, E. (1992) *Organizational culture and leadership*, San Franscisco, CA: Jossey Bass.

Schein, E. (2004) *Organizational culture and leadership* (3rd edn), San Franscisco, CA: Jossey Bass.

Schein, V., Mueller, R., Lituchy, T. and Liu, J. (1996) 'Think manager – think male: a global phenomenon?', *Journal of Organizational Behavior*, 17 (1), 33–41.

Scott, T., Mannion, R., Davies, H. and Marshall, M. (2003) 'Implementing culture change in health care: theory and practice', *International Journal for Quality in Health Care*, 15 (2), 111–18.

Scott, W.R. (2001) *Institutions and organizations*, Thousand Oaks, CA: Sage.

Selznick, P. (1957) *Leadership in administration*, Evanston, IL: Row Peterson.

Senge, P. (1994) *The fifth discipline*, New York: Doubleday.

Shamir, B., Pillai, R., Bligh, M. and Uhl-Bien, M. (2007) *Follower-centred perspectives on leadership*, Greenwich, CT: IAP Publishing.

Sheaff, R., Rogers, A., Pickard, S., Marshall, M., Campbell, S., Sibbald, B., Halliwell, S. and Roland, M. (2003) 'A subtle governance: "soft" medical leadership in English primary care', *Sociology of Health and Illness*, 25, 408–28.

Shipton, H., Armstrong, C., West, M. and Dawson, J. (2008) 'The impact of leadership and quality climate on hospital performance', *International Journal for Quality in Health Care*, 20 (6), 439–45, published online 10 September.

Simpson, J. (2008) *The politics of leadership*, London: Leading Edge Publications.

Sinclair, A. (2005) *Doing leadership differently: Gender, power and sexuality in a changing business culture*, Melbourne: Melbourne University Press.

Smircich, L. and Morgan, G. (1982) 'Leadership: the management of meaning', *Journal of Applied Behavioral Science*, 18 (3), 257–73.

Sosik, J. (2006) 'Full range leadership', in R. Burke and C. Cooper (eds) *Inspiring leadership*, London: Routledge.

Souba, W. (2004) 'New ways of understanding and accomplishing leadership in academic medicine', *Journal of Surgical Research*, 117 (2), 177–86.

Souba, W. and Day, D. (2006) 'Leadership values in academic medicine', *Academic Medicine*, 81 (1), 20–6.

Sparrow, P. (2000) 'Strategic management in a world turned upside-down: the role of cognition, intuition and emotional intelligence', in P. Flood, S. Carroll, L. Gorman and T. Dromgoole (eds) *Managing strategic implementation*, Oxford: Blackwell.

Spillane, J. (2005) 'Distributed leadership', *The Educational Forum*, 69 (2), 143–50.

Stewart, J. (2001) *Modernizing government*, Basingstoke: Palgrave Macmillan.

Stogdill, R. (1950) 'Leadership, membership and organization', *Psychological Bulletin*, 47, 1–14.

Stogdill, R. (1974) *Handbook of leadership: A survey of theory and research*, New York: Free Press.

Stoker, G. (2006) 'Public value management: a new narrative for networked governance?', *American Review of Public Administration*, 36 (1), 41–57.

Stordeur, S., D'Hoore, W. and Vandenberghe, C. (2001) 'Leadership, organizational stress, and emotional exhaustion among hospital nursing staff', *Journal of Advanced Nursing*, 35 (4), 533–42.

Storey, J. (2004) *Leadership in organizations: Current issues and key trends*, London: Routledge.

Taunton, R.L., Boyle, D.K., Woods, C., Hansen, H. and Bott, M. (1997) 'Manager leadership and retention of hospital staff nurses', *Western Journal of Nursing Research*, 19 (2), 205–26.

Tavanti, M. (2008) 'Transactional leadership', in A. Marturano and J. Gosling (eds) *Leadership: The key concepts*, London: Routledge.

Tichy, N. and Cohen, E. (1997) *The leadership engine: How winning companies build leaders at every level*, New York: Harper Collins.

Tilley, N. (2010) 'Can public leadership be evaluated?' in S. Brookes and K. Grint (eds) *The public leadership challenge*, London: Palgrave.

Tranfield, D., Denyer, D. and Smart, P. (2003) 'Towards a methodology for developing evidence-based management knowledge by means of systematic reviews', *British Journal of Management*, 14, 207–22.

Tritter, J. (2010) 'Framing the production of health in terms of public value', in J. Benington and J. Moore (eds) *Public value: Theory and practice*, Basingstoke: Palgrave Macmillan.

Uhl-Bien, M. and Marion, R. (2009) 'Complexity leadership in bureaucratic forms of organizing: a meso model', *Leadership Quarterly*, 20, 631–50.

Vandenberghe, C., Stordeur, S. and D'hoore, W. (2002) 'Transactional and transformational leadership in nursing: structural validity and substantive relationships', *European Journal of Psychological Assessment*, 18 (1), 16–29.

Walshe, K. and Rundall, T. (2001) 'Evidence-based management: from theory to practice in health care', *Milbank Quarterly*, 79 (3), 429–58.

Walshe, K., Harvey, G., Hyde, P. and Pandit, N. (2004) 'Organizational failure and turnaround: lessons for public services from the for-profit sector', *Public Money and Management*, 24 (4), 201–8.

Weick, K. (1995) *Sense-making in organizations*, Thousand Oaks, CA: Sage.

Weick, K.L., Prydun, M. and Walsh, T. (2002) 'What the emerging workforce wants in its leaders', *Journal of Nursing Scholarship*, 34 (3), 283–8.

Weiner, B., Shortell, S. and Alexander, J. (1997) 'Promoting clinical involvement in hospital quality improvement efforts: the effects of top management, board and physician leadership', *Health Services Research*, 32 (4), 491–510.

West, M., Borrill, C., Dawson, J., Brodbeck, F., Shapiro, D. and Haward, B. (2003) 'Leadership clarity and team innovation in health care', *Leadership Quarterly*, 14, 393–410.

Westley, F. and Mintzberg, H. (1989) 'Visionary leadership and strategic management', *Strategic Management Journal*, 10, 17–32.

Wheatley, M. (1992) *Leadership and the new science*, San Francisco, CA: Berrett-Koehler.

Willcocks, S. (2005) 'Doctors and leadership in the UK National Health Service', *Clinician in Management*, 13, 11–21.

Williams, S. (2004a) *Literature review: Evidence of the role of leadership and leadership development in contributing to the effectiveness of major IT-led transformation*, London: NHS Leadership Centre.

Williams, S. (2004b) *Literature review: Evidence of the contribution leadership development for professional groups makes in driving their organisations forward*, Henley: Henley Management College.

Wright, K., Rowitz, L., Merkle, A., Reid, M., Robinson, G., Herzog, B., Weber, D., Carmichael, D., Balderson, T. and Baker, E. (2000) 'Competency development in public health leadership', *American Journal of Public Health*, 90 (8), 1202–7.

Yammarino, F. (1994) 'Indirect leadership: transformational leadership at a distance', in B. Bass and B. Avolio (eds) *Improving organizational effectiveness through transformational leadership*, Thousand Oaks, CA: Sage.

Yukl, G. (2006) *Leadership in organizations* (6th edn), Upper Saddle River, NJ: Pearson Prentice Hall.

Yukl, G. (2009) 'Leading organizational learning: reflections on theory and research', *Leadership Quarterly*, 20, 49–53.

Zaleznik, A. (1977) 'Managers and leaders: are they different?', *Harvard Business Review*, 55, 67–78.

Index

Note: Page numbers followed by *fig* and *tab* refer to information in a figure or a table.

A

Aarons, G.A. 104
academic literature *see* evidence base for leadership
activities and consequences of leadership 101, 103-5
adaptability as meta-competency 84*tab*
adaptive leadership 20, 33, 91
  and challenges 58-60, 73, 120
  and context 40-1, 46-7
  and innovation 70
'adaptive' problems *see* 'wicked' (adaptive) problems
Alexander, J. 64-6, 84-5
Alford, J. 106
Alimo-Metcalfe, B. 17, 87, 114, 119
Allison, M. 15, 17
American Organization of Nurse Executives 67-8
Arnold, K. 104
attributional error and research 80, 96-7, 109
authority
  formal and informal leadership 26-8, 37
  and position 17-18, 35-6
Avolio, B.J. 88-9

B

Bailey, C. 47-8, 102
balanced scorecard evaluation 107-8, 109
Barling, J. 104, 121-2
Barrett, L. 105
Bass, B. 16, 76, 87, 88, 89
Bate, P. 106
behaviour theory 10, 16, 75, 77-84, 92
Benington, J. 41, 46, 58, 59, 99-100, 117, 121
Bennis, W. 17
big picture sense-making 51, 53-4, 72, 129-30

black and minority ethnic (BME) managers 91
Blackler, F. 44, 60-1
boards and capabilities 86
Bolden, R. 80
Borrill, C. 103
Boyatzis, R. 77-8, 79*fig*, 80
Boyne, G. 67
Brazier, D. 47
Briscoe, J. 83
Bryan, K. 20, 30, 34-5
Bryman, A. 16-17, 18, 33, 91
Buchanan, D. 19, 41, 107-8
Burdett Trust for Nursing 86
bureaucratic organisations 47
Burke, R. 17, 33, 121
Burns, J. 1, 14, 16, 87, 88
Burr, J. 47-8, 102

C

Cabinet Office: Performance and Innovation Unit 3, 96
capabilities of leadership 7*fig*, 9-10, 75-93, 127
  behaviours and competencies 77-84, 92
  capability models 122
  and leadership development 10-11, 121-2, 125
  for leading networks and teams 84-6, 92
  public value perspective 101
  traits for leaders 76-7, 92
  use of term 78
capacity building 33, 44, 115
  consequences of leadership 105
  nurturing future leaders 66*tab*, 72, 73, 89
  turnaround strategies 67, 73
  see also human capital; social capital
challenges of leadership 7*fig*, 9, 51-73, 127, 128
  in healthcare 4, 51

Lightning Source UK Ltd.
Milton Keynes UK
UKOW01f0034211017
311371UK00003B/132/P